New Advances in Magnetic Resonance Imaging

Edited by Denis Larrivee

Published in London, United Kingdom

New Advances in Magnetic Resonance Imaging
http://dx.doi.org/10.5772/intechopen.111259
Edited by Denis Larrivee

Contributors
Pilar Giraldo Castellano, Mercedes Roca Espiau, Jorge Rolando Ortiz, Juliana Gonzalez, Juan Sebastian Herrera, Mahi L. Ashwath, Hunter Frederiksen, Corina Iorgoveanu, Naima Amin, Muhammad Yousaf, Karima Hami, Aron Hernandez-Trinidad, Teodoro Cordova-Fraga, Rafael Guzman-Cabrera, Blanca Olivia Murillo-Ortiz, Denis Larrivee

First published in London, United Kingdom, 2024 by IntechOpen
IntechOpen is the global imprint of INTECHOPEN LIMITED, registered in England and Wales, registration number: 11086078, 5 Princes Gate Court, London, SW7 2QJ, United Kingdom

British Library Cataloguing-in-Publication Data
A catalogue record for this book is available from the British Library

Additional hard and PDF copies can be obtained from orders@intechopen.com

New Advances in Magnetic Resonance Imaging
Edited by Denis Larrivee
p. cm.
Print ISBN 978-1-83769-192-0
Online ISBN 978-1-83769-193-7
eBook (PDF) ISBN 978-1-83769-194-4

For EU product safety concerns:
IN TECH d.o.o., Prolaz Marije Krucifikse Kozulić 3, 51000 Rijeka, Croatia,
info@intechopen.com or visit our website at intechopen.com.

Meet the editor

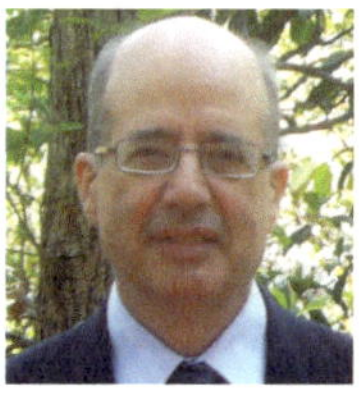

Dr. Denis Larrivee is a visiting scholar at the Mind and Brain Institute, University of Navarra Medical School and Loyola University, Chicago. He has held professorships at the Weill Cornell University Medical College, NYC, and Purdue University, Indiana. A former fellow at Yale University's Medical School, Dr. Larrivee received the Association for Research in Vision and Ophthalmology's first-place award for studies on photoreceptor degenerative and developmental mechanisms. He is the editor of seven books on clinical neuroscience and neurotechnology and an editorial board member of the *Annals of Neurology and Neurological Sciences* (USA) and *EC Neurology* (UK). He is also the author of more than 100 papers and book chapters in such journals as *Neurology and Neurological Sciences, Journal of Neuroscience, Frontiers in Human Neuroscience, Journal of Religion and Mental Health*, and *IEEE Xplore*. In 2018, he was a finalist for the international Joseph Ratzinger Expanded Reason Award sponsored by the Francis Vittorio University of Madrid.

Contents

Preface

Magnetic resonance imaging (MRI) is one of the most widely employed technologies for the clinical imaging of soft tissues due to its high contrast and spatial resolution, absence of ionizing radiation, and the current breadth of methodological applications. Much of the present diagnostic power of MRI is due to the technology's reliance on the nuclear magnetic moment of hydrogen and its manner of detection. Hydrogen is abundant in soft tissues and possesses a readily detectable magnetic moment in the presence of an externally applied magnetic field. Technical details for generating the field trace their origin to Bloch and Purcell's original method of demonstrating the nuclear magnetic phenomenon. In their technique, the interaction between the nuclear magnetic moment and the magnetic field generated a resonance frequency that was electronically detected by an inducting coil. In its clinical usage, a linear gradient was introduced in the magnetic field, enabling the resonance frequency to be varied as a function of its position along the gradient. This permitted the sampling of biological tissue via a Fourier space along a single axis one point at a time. Measurement of the signal with respect to phase differences along a second axis provided a unique set of values corresponding to each xy set of coordinates on the tissue plane.

This basic technological approach has since provided sufficient latitude to permit the wide-ranging evolution that has led to today's generation of MRI applications. A small sampling includes such well-established procedures as parallel imaging, which has substantially lessened the long acquisition intervals plaguing early clinical use; computational algorithms for preprocessing steps of co-registration and denoising, which are now routine; and functional MRI for brain activity, currently used widely in clinical research.

New advances are benefiting from a synergy of the current procedures together with the parallel evolution now occurring in the computational disciplines. Among the factors propelling the development of functional approaches, for example, are the currently evolved capabilities for rapid data acquisition, enhanced detection, and improved physiological models of function, which together underpin the growing trend toward monitoring dynamic properties in an increasingly data-driven, large-scale computational environment. Structural analyses are also undergoing a significant evolution. While MRI has traditionally been used chiefly for structural tissue determinations, the difficulties in managing the burgeoning wealth of imagery data are increasingly requiring computational processing prior to examination by clinicians. Upcoming trends to address this need include new algorithms with enhanced computational power for feature extraction and pattern recognition. Computational developments also include specialized procedures that handle big data analyses, such as MRI fingerprinting and whole brain dynamics.

The current text presents select cases of how these trends are being incorporated into a new generation of MRI applications. The introductory chapter, Chapter 1, covers the current capabilities, providing a foundation for how the next generation of applications will benefit from knowledge previously gained in these standard areas.

The book's focus then shifts to how the current capabilities are incorporated in three domains that are experiencing especially rapid growth: functional and dynamic imaging in cardiac health and disease, advances in computational machine learning and its application to brain networks, and multiparametric, tissue-specific procedures.

Dynamic MRI in Cardiovascular Diagnosis

Cardiac MRI (CMR) currently offers precise visualization of myocardial tissue structure and function that has proven to be critical for assessing cardiovascular disease. Chapter 2 describes the current broad range of CMR techniques and discusses how a similar range of next-generation applications are building on these abilities. The latter include, for example, updated structural mapping techniques that provide a comprehensive analysis and image of the entire heart with single scans for improved detection of fibrosis and edema that are often missed on older scanning procedures. Novel cardiac methods also include procedures for estimating cardiac tissue strain, obtained using the procedures of displacement encoding with stimulated echocardiography (DENSE) and feature tracking (FT), a post-processing algorithm that calculates myocardial deformation.

Improvements in the management of patients with congenital heart disease have significantly increased the number of patients surviving well into adulthood. Long-term care for such patients requires ongoing follow-up to detect and treat long-term complications. Chapter 3 describes an MRI procedure that measures four-dimensional heart flow in congenital patients. Four-dimensional flow allows a velocity assessment of the whole heart and major vessels with electrocardiogram gating and can be taken in a single acquisition. This is especially relevant for complex heart diagnoses. As one of multiple examples, it can assess the kinetic energy of blood flow, which provides a diagnostic measure for determining ventricular efficiency.

Machine Learning and Brain Network Analysis Methods for MRI

The rapidly increasing volume of MRI data generated by new MRI procedures underscores the imperative for computational resources and serves to drive the development of computational capabilities in virtually all stages of MRI analysis, from acquisition and preprocessing to image reconstruction and feature extraction, and to big data issues. This has resulted in the current proliferation of machine learning methods that have enhanced image acquisition, analysis, and clinical decision-making. Chapter 4 provides a theoretical background for these methods and reviews how various applications are used in specific MRI stages. The chapter discusses, for example, convolutional neural networks, which have proven highly effective for image classification. Advanced computational analysis is of particular benefit for complex functional analyses, such as those employed in analyzing brain networks. Such computational procedures are increasingly applied to functional studies of brain activity.

Functional MRI (fMRI) of the quiescent brain, notably, has revealed that brain activity is highly organized into a group of brain networks (RSNs). Designated resting state, functional, magnetic resonance imaging (RS-fMRI), the method is currently the most powerful tool available for assessing the functional connectivity properties of brain networks. Chapter 5 discusses recent developments in RS-fMRI that seek to build on such functional connectivity determinations by relating causal sources of connectivity changes to brain states and behavior. Coupled with new modeling procedures, these determinations provide insight into dynamic brain topology and its relationship to brain states. Because of the large amounts of data generated by these studies, traditional data-driven methods for handling RS-fMRI data, such as independent components analysis and graph theoretic approaches, become unwieldy and lose descriptive power at elevated data levels. The chapter describes, among several other topics, current efforts to address big data handling that can be used to accurately gauge network structure and dynamics.

Multiparametric, Tissue-Specific MRI Procedures

Among MRI's imaging capabilities is a capacity for distinguishing compositional differences and anomalies in different tissues. This is increasingly used to advantage in the determination of the many diseases affecting bone tissue. Normal bone always contains both fat and red marrow, and these undergo variations in fatty composition/hematopoietic cellularity as part of a transformation phenomenon associated with these diseases. Marrow fat is distinguished by an elevated signal intensity due to its high proton content, whereas hematopoietic marrow has a much smaller signal. Using magnetic resonance spectroscopy, it is possible to quantify these differences, which enables a precise determination of changes occurring within the bone cavity.

Chapter 6 describes these advanced MRI procedures and their use in a wide range of major bone diseases and other clinical entities. New advances in magnetic field strength, gradient strength, and coils have enabled the development of novel pulse sequences, which have transformed knee MRI from a routine procedure of tissue structure to one of ultrastructure and even postoperative ligament reconstructions, which has previously constituted a challenge. Chapter 7 discusses these advanced procedures for finely delineating knee tissue structure. For example, isotropic three-dimensional MRI permits thin-slice MRI with a spatial resolution of less than 1 mm and is seen in oblique planes, which help analyze complex structures like static and dynamic knee stabilizers. Enhanced three-dimensional visualization from various angles is expected to assist preoperative planning and achieve better clinical outcomes in patients with difficult-to-treat ligament and meniscal injuries.

Diagnostic analyses have traditionally benefitted from studies exploring pulse sequences that optimize image features while minimizing artifact contributions and scanning time. The introduction of non-linear gradients, for example, was undertaken to improve image quality in highly undersampled MRI. Protocols for assessing pulse sequences are of interest for their utility in determining preferred sequences. Chapter 8 presents a pre-diagnostic protocol for assessing sequences that optimize these basic relationships. As a proof-of-principle demonstration, the procedure examines three frequently used pulse sequences: Fast Spin Echo (FSE), Fast Fluid Attenuated Inversion Recovery (FLAIR), and Conventional Spin Echo (CSE).

Denis Larrivee
Mind and Brain Institute,
University of Navarra Medical School,
Pamplona, Spain

Section 1

Introduction

Chapter 1

Introductory Chapter: New Advances in MRI Clinical Analysis

Denis Larrivee

1. Introduction

1.1 Detecting the nuclear magnetic moment

While magnetic resonance imaging has been used clinically since the early 1980s [1], the development of the technique traces its origin to Bloch and Purcell's demonstration of the nuclear magnetic phenomenon several decades earlier [2, 3]. Their work showed that in the presence of a constant magnetic field, nuclear magnetic moments generated a resonance frequency that could be electronically detected by means of an inducting coil. The ability to detect an electrical signal induced by the magnetic moment made possible the development of adjunct procedures for spatially profiling analytical specimens. Advances in MRI that have since propelled its clinical application have built on the physical principles underlying the magnetic moment and its detection used in the Bloch and Purcell demonstrations.

A key factor in the clinical use of the nuclear magnetic moment is the quantum mechanical effect present in hydrogen protons, which are abundant in soft tissue and confer the equivalent of an angular "spin" on the nucleus [4]. In the presence of an externally applied magnetic field, the magnetic moment generated by the spin processes about the axis of the applied field at a rate proportional to the external field and at a fixed angle to the field's axis, which defines the Larmor frequency. Within the static field, a second, perpendicular magnetic field applied by radiofrequency can excite the processing nuclear moment, changing the energy level and frequency of the magnetic moment with respect to the static field. In practice, this second field is applied in pulses typically lasting on the order of microseconds. Energy input from the pulses is then re-emitted between pulses as the magnetic moment returns to equilibrium, a process termed free induction decay. Relaxation to thermal equilibrium can occur either longitudinally, with loss of energy to the surrounding environment (a reduction in signal intensity, termed T_1), or transversely, with energy exchange (but not loss) with neighboring nuclei (seen in a broadening of signal phase, termed T_2). T_1 and T_2 values are defined as the lengths of time taken for their respective signals to decline by 63% (or to 37% from the equilibrium value), which adopt first order, exponential decay.

1.2 Spatial resolution and localization

Although the measured signal has its origin in the physical features inherent to the tissue, its detection and subsequent conversion to an anatomical image relies on technical features that amplify, resolve, and reconstruct the unique spatial and physical properties of the image [5]. Localization of the tissue signal, notably, requires the use of magnetic field gradients, which is achieved by varying the static field strength during signal retrieval. In a typical application, the gradient introduces a linear variation in the static field strength along a tissue axis. Because spin precession frequency is directly proportional to field strength, there is a one-to-one correspondence between frequency and position. Gradients can assume any orthogonal direction and, in principle, can be used to reconstruct 3-dimensional images.

Faster or slower precession, and so higher and lower frequency, is detected as a higher or lower signal. Accordingly, manipulating the magnitude of the field strength range modulates the range of frequencies emitted for signal retrieval along a single axis. Imaging data acquired with small gradients has a small frequency range, limiting the frequency differential that can cover a pixel and so also limiting resolution. Larger gradients expand the frequency range, increasing resolution. When plotted, low frequencies are thus distributed centrally and high frequencies peripherally in a mathematical domain termed K-space [6, 7]; all image points thereby contain information from all frequencies. Planar localization requires encoding information along a second axis, a process also achieved by means of a static field gradient, but in which the phase difference along the second axis is monitored. Because phase differences can only be detected with respect to a reference value, a single scan is required for each phase encoded value. Information from both axes must then be mathematically transformed (by Fourier transform) to yield an x-y, planar image.

Because the typical and early use of the method—termed spin echo—sequentially varied the strength of the static field gradient, an important limitation in the use of MRI imaging has been the scanning time required to produce an adequately resolved image. Scanning time is a function of two factors: the interval between radiofrequency pulses, termed repetition time (TR), and the number of scans required for phase encoding and detection. The product of these yields the total scan time. Employing this protocol, typical scanning times could take on the order of minutes to hours, with higher resolution images needing longer intervals and so corresponding corrections for time related artifacts such as patient movement. Because of such artifacts, scanning time has posed a significant obstacle to image acquisition and quality.

1.3 Evolution in MRI procedures

Much of the early evolution in MRI methods thus sought to achieve a balance between data acquisition procedures that provided for sufficient spatial and temporal resolution and contrast and the time required to achieve a desired image. An example of this balancing is seen in the line reductions first introduced to the basic spin echo protocol [6]. A drawback to this approach, however, was the attendant loss in either resolution or image size due to the loss of frequency information. In the fast spin, echo planar or multi echo approach, for example, scanning time was reduced by taking multiple lines after the radio frequency pulse. A chief disadvantage of this latter approach, however, was the rapid loss in signal strength due to energy transferal during T2 acquisition, permitting only 3–4 lines per RF pulse, with significant deterioration in image quality.

While the objectives of reducing acquisition time and achieving enhanced spatial and temporal resolution have been of perennial interest in MRI development, new developments for addressing these and other objectives have in turn revealed new needs that invited corresponding solutions. The widespread use of parallel imaging [8], for example, was due to its ability to accelerate data acquisition while maintaining high resolution through reductions in phase encoding lines and the use of algorithms that corrected subsampling aliasing. Such rapid acquisition methods led to the proliferation of multi-parametric approaches, which then facilitated quantification studies for MR fingerprinting [9]. These, and extended MR functional analyses, for instance, whole brain resting state fMRI [10], have engendered the further development of big data methods for the accompanying computational requirements, while data processing needs for processes such as feature extraction [11] propelled the use of machine learning to reduce diagnostic load. Indeed, the range of new techniques extends from advances in image acquisition to data processing and inference to computation and data handling, enhanced spatial resolution, and functional analyses. To illustrate the current proliferation, this introductory chapter to New Advances in Magnetic Resonance Imaging presents a select representation of techniques that trace their evolution from the physical and detection principles first identified by Bloch and Purcell. Chapters that follow each present a single, recently evolved MRI technique in greater detail. It is hoped that the novelty of these advances will be a source of inspiration for the engaged professional and interested scientist alike.

2. Acquisition procedures: advances in parallel imaging

Parallel imaging is now used in nearly every clinical MRI scan for rapid data acquisition, for numerous reasons [8]. Many abdominal and cardiac scans, for example, are taken with patients holding their breath, with its obvious need for short scanning times. In other cases, for instance, multiline sequences following excitation pulses (e.g., in turbo spin echo), blurring artifacts are introduced due to the substantial T2 decay occurring during line retrieval. In still other applications, rapid data acquisition is essential because of the need to acquire large data sets [12, 13].

In parallel imaging, scanning time is reduced because the phased array coils yield unique views of the tissue objective, eliminating the scanning time for a significant portion of the region subject to gradient encoding [8, 14]. Due to the rapid decline in sensitivity of each coil element with increasing distance from the coil, this limits data acquisition to a clearly delineated, tissue profile. Individual images are combined to yield a comprehensive image. As a matter of principle, the maximum acceleration factor is related to the number of coils. Since most parallel imaging often employs 4–8 coil arrays and arrays containing 32, or even 128, channels are known (e.g., cardiac imaging), the reduction in scan time can be substantial.

Protocols for parallel imaging are currently classed according to whether aliased pixels are segregated in the imaging domain (SENSitivity Encoding or SENSE) or in K-space (Generalized Autocalibrating Partial Parallel Acquisition or GRAPPA) [14]. Techniques that act on the image domain first reconstruct and then correct, while those that act on the frequency domain first correct and then reconstruct. For those segregating in the imaging domain, prior knowledge of the coil sensitivity profiles enables separation of folded pixels from the undersampled image to recover the full image. Recent improvements have included phase-constrained SENSE. Whereas in conventional SENSE unknown variables are complex value, in phase-constrained SENSE, values are real, reducing the variable number by half. In contrast to the SENSE techniques, the GRAPPA algorithm is a K-space technique, which operates on acquired frequency information that is embedded in K-space. The technique is based on the principle that K-space information is shared between points in K-space due to the variation in multiple static field gradients; hence, missing information can be computationally reconstructed from acquired K-space data. In order to reconstruct information from the missing points, acquired data points must be adjusted by weighting using an autocalibration signal obtained from another region of K-space.

Two recent modifications of the GRAPPA technique have included the 2D CAIPIRINHA and Wave-CAIPI techniques [15]. In 2D CAIPIRINHA, acceleration in the K_y and K_z directions is accompanied by a phase offset along K_z. This generates unique frequency patterns that require less computational resources for resolving aliasing. The Wave-CAIPI technique builds on 2D CAIPIRINHA by adding sinusoidal gradients along the K_y and K_z axes with a 180° shift. These additions amplify the acceleration by a factor of 9 over the 2D CAIPIRINHA technique. Unlike other very fast acquisitions, Wave-CAIPI is not subject to blurring from data gridding or artifacts from distortion due to uneven static magnetic fields.

3. Reconstruction procedures for image analysis

The initial stages of image acquisition, preprocessing, and segmentation prepare the data for extraction of meaningful information. By definition, these steps involve removal of nonmeaningful or noise-based signals. One common source of noise, for example, is due to patient movement. Motion artifacts are corrected by registering sequential images, which can be carried out using available algorithms suited for medical imaging. A current standard for MRI image registration is the InsightToolKit (ITK), which contains a suite of algorithms including such processes as transformations, similarity metrics, and contrast normalization [11].

Recent trends in preprocessing and segmentation (e.g., denoising) have employed machine-based learning applications. Due to the labor involved, another major trend in machine-based learning procedures has been that of feature recognition and classification [16]. The high quantity of imaging data acquired from existing MRI scanning, especially, has made clinical diagnoses based on MRI images increasingly laborious, driving efforts for automated data abstraction and analysis. Computationally, machine learning relies on algorithms derived from neural network structures, which are composed of nodes joined by weighted edges. Inputs to nodes are weighted by a set of parameters and multiplied by transfer functions, for example, sigmoid and hyperbolic tangent functions, which transform weighted inputs. Among the most widely used of these deep neural networks (DNN) are the convolutional neural network (CNN), ResNet, the generative adversarial neural networks (GANs), and the U-nets.

Deep network models used for processing whole images are highly complicated, which significantly amplifies the processing time. For example, a CNN training model can often create millions of parameters in searches for feature classification. This drawback has been addressed by the use of image representations of smaller size that increases the processing efficiency. Most current feature extraction applications utilize wavelet transformation techniques in conjunction with neural network processing for MRI images [17]. The wavelet transform is used to remove extraneous detail and make the image more efficient for network processing; hence, approximated images have denser information content than original images. Convolutional layers then apply an initial filtering to produce an initial feature map, that is, what the network deems as unique features, which is refined by further network processing.

4. Multi-information sourcing

Compared to methods for single parameter data analysis, models using multi-parametric techniques offer the chief advantage of assessing correlations between multiple quantitative parameters of interest [9], with the potential for significantly greater accuracy. Various relevant MRI quantities include, but are not limited to, longitudinal (T1) and transverse (T2) relaxation times as well as retrospective synthesis of conventional MR contrasts, which are monitored in conjunction with novel techniques for rapid data acquisition and computational analysis.

Multi-parametric, analytical techniques currently employ similar strategies [18] with simultaneous sampling of the parameter and K-spaces, in which transient-state data are obtained by varying the acquisition parameters and undersampled K-space snapshots are taken after each excitation. Parametric maps are then computed using a physical model *via* the Bloch equations. Several procedures that have evolved from this approach include magnetic resonance fingerprinting (MRF) [18] and quantitative transient-state imaging (QTI).

In MRF, modulating the MRI sequence parameters across the time domain yields a time series of weighted MRI images, with each tissue having a unique MRI signal fingerprint. Such fingerprints can be computationally simulated and a dictionary of tissue specific fingerprints built from the simulations. During image reconstruction, putative fingerprints are matched to this dictionary. The fingerprint with the greatest correlation in the dictionary provides the MRI parameters for a given voxel. After all voxels are analyzed, parametric maps are then constructed. Due to its ability to recognize very specific structural elements, MRF has the potential for diagnosis of a wide variety of clinical conditions [19–22]. Novel techniques like quantitative sequencing enable clinical approaches capable of accelerated quantitative mapping of dynamic physiological processes. For example, such techniques have been used to examine blood flow, with computation made of velocity scalars or vectors that could be employed in cardiac assessments. In one study, computations of scalar velocities were computed in a direction perpendicular to a vessel slice based on multi-parametric T_1, T_2, and proton density recordings [23]. A drawback to such methods is that of their reliance on physical models of the physiological events the quantitative mapping is intended to simulate, with the potential for loss of valuable data. Moreover, the complexity of such models can demand increasing computational resources, significantly extending the data acquisition period.

5. Functional approaches using MRI

Blood oxygenation-dependent contrast, termed BOLD or fMRI imaging [24], was developed to indirectly assess neural activity in the brain by monitoring activity-induced changes in blood oxygenation. BOLD exploits the neurovascular mechanism of hyperemia, whereby localized brain activity recruits increased blood oxygenation within the region of activation. In typically used protocols, the image sequence relies on T2* weighting with scan times under 5 seconds to measure the hemodynamic response function. Since its discovery, use of this procedure has undergone extraordinary growth [13, 24].

The dependence of the BOLD signal on neurovascular mechanisms, however, has meant that fMRI is also constrained by limitations inherent in the hemodynamic response. Chief among these is the much slower response time than the underlying neural processes being measured. Temporal information of spiking events is therefore heavily blurred, requiring the use of mathematical processing, like that of the general linear model or experimental block protocols, to infer event related, signal activity [24]. With processing, temporal resolution in the 100 ms range can be achieved, which is roughly tenfold slower than the neural events being monitored.

5.1 High-strength imaging

Another challenge to fMRI is that of the low signal to noise ratio (SNR), a consequence of data acquisition, and constraints limiting the extent of preprocessing that can be performed. One of the technical improvements now being attempted to improve the SNR is the use of high-strength magnetic fields, which enhances the anatomical specificity of imaging. Whereas most scanning is done using 3 T fields, equipment using 7 T fields is becoming increasingly prevalent. At these higher field strengths, it has been shown that less spatial smoothing is required and neural activity in cases of resting state networks displays higher correlation coefficients, indicating greater spatial resolution [25–27]. On the other hand, use of higher field strengths has several drawbacks, including longer sampling intervals, inhomogeneous magnetic field properties, and the logarithmic growth in specific absorption rate (SAR) with increasing field strength [28, 29].

5.2 Multimodal studies (w EEG/MEG)

Among the techniques used to overcome the temporal limitations of fMRI have been multimodal approaches, which combine fMRI with such methods as the EEG or MEG. Both EEG and MEG display rapid temporal responses, with the capability for resolving neural events at millisecond scales. Use of these approaches in conjunction with fMRI is thus premised on the greatly improved temporal resolution offered by these procedures. Advanced technologies have now been developed to simultaneously record EEG and fMRI signal, which help to understand the relationship between the spatial and temporal characteristics of physiological signals [30]. Nonetheless, in comparison to fMRI alone, combined approaches have seen limited use. In the case of EEG, spatial resolution is greatly inferior to that of fMRI and MEG approaches that suffer from source localization issues. This means that the experimental design or clinical assessment must clearly attribute the signal sources prior to drawing experimental and/or clinical conclusions in such combined approaches.

5.3 DIANA fMRI

The persistence of interpretive difficulties with multimodal approaches has generated a long-standing interest in the development of alternative methods capable of both high spatial and temporal resolution. One recently developed method has merged the detection of ultra-weak magnetic fields generated by neural electrical activity with the fMRI detection of the hemodynamic response [31]. This approach, termed Direct Imaging of Neuronal Activity for functional MRI (DIANA-fMRI), interleaves K-space lines used for imaging the hemodynamic response with a K-space line that directly measures the ultra-weak magnetic field. Millisecond resolution is achieved using fast, low-angle shot (FLASH); gradient-echo imaging; and short repetition intervals (e.g., 5 ms). When carried out at high field strengths (9.4 Tesla), signal to noise ratios are reported to be in the range of 20 to 1. To date, the technique has been used only on animal models.

While promising, the technique suffers from its own unique set of interpretive uncertainties. For example, electromagnetic effects based on neuronal current models appear to be ruled out as these oppose the direction of the observed DIANA response. Moreover, in humans, increasing the stimulus duration does not lead to correlative signal changes, suggesting that the signal may be confounded by other interactions such as inflow effects and subject motion. These uncertainties suggest that further development of the approach will require improved understanding of the biophysical factors contributing to the DIANA signal.

5.4 Resting state fMRI

One of the most significant fMRI developments is the use of fMRI during rest, coined resting state-fMRI (RS-fMRI). RS-fMRI focuses on spontaneous low-frequency fluctuations (< 0.1 Hz) in the BOLD signal that occur in the absence of task-related activities. The functional significance of these fluctuations was first recognized by Biswal et al. [32] in a study in which subjects were told not to perform any cognitive, language, or motor tasks. After determining the correlation between the BOLD time course of a seed region identified by bilateral finger tapping and that of all other areas in the brain, the authors found that fluctuations in the left somatosensory cortex were highly correlated with homologous areas in the contralateral hemisphere. This observed correlation led to their conclusion that such "resting networks" manifested the functional connectivity of the brain. The observation of spontaneous, synchronous fluctuations occurring between brain regions has since led to studies that have identified as many as 7 to 17 other stable networks [33], with 7 consistently agreed upon.

Because characterization of resting state networks (RSNs) in the human brain relies on the analysis of temporal fluctuations in the blood oxygenation level-dependent (BOLD) signal, the delineation of RSNs has been directly dependent on the ability of fMRI to detect neural activity [6]. The dependence on the BOLD signal means that RS-fMRI shares advantages that accrue to fMRI—the ability to monitor neural activity, albeit indirectly—as well as disadvantages that characterize its use. Chief among these limitations is fMRI's temporal resolution, which is dependent on the hemodynamic response time [34]. Accordingly, a key factor in the use of RS-fMRI is the measurement of neural activity fluctuations rather than spiking events per se.

Early studies of RSN functional connectivities, like that of Biswal et al. [32, 35], relied on the selection of regions of interest based on investigator preferences. However, while the simplicity and interpretability of the ROI technique make it procedurally facile and a frequently adopted approach, the method relies entirely on user-defined ROIs and so is limited for network discovery by its a priori, selected criteria. Due to this caveat and coupled with the evolution of mathematical models and improved computational capabilities, there has been a paradigm shift from that of imposing initial conditions on the data to that of extracting patterns of brain activity directly from the raw time series. The main example of this approach is independent component analysis [36]. In this approach, the time series signal is assumed to be due to multiple spatiotemporal processes that are statistically independent of each other. By extracting the independent signals, various time courses of specific brain regions can be constructed and grouped into maps representative of their spatial distribution. Another approach to the interpretation of RS-fMRI datasets employs graph theory, where activity sources comprise nodes and connectivity defines the edges that link these nodes [10, 36]. Unlike ICA, which focuses chiefly on the strength of correlation between different domains, graph theory characterizes the features of network topology. The graph theory approach describes the interaction between nodes by means of such graph parameters as average path length, clustering coefficients, node degree, centrality measures, and level of modularity. Graph theory is thus a promising technique for exploring the integration and segregation of networks in the brain. Among the topological features studied, modularity, the assessment of the presence of functionally independent units or modules that compose resting state networks, has increasingly been used to characterize functional adjustments occurring during behavior, network perturbations, or pathologies that affect network function, revealing significant alterations in such pathologies as stroke [37] and psychiatric disease [38, 39].

In principle, inferences of causality from directed functional connectivity determinations can be extended to brain-wide neuronal dynamics. Empirical studies from RS-fMRI, for example, show that RSNs are differentiated on the basis of their metastability and synchrony [40]. These and similar observations have led to models of brain function and behavior that predict that the human brain at rest operates at maximum metastability, that is, in a state of maximal network switching. The demonstration of RSN properties like metastability thus suggests that directed connectivity changes may be used to assess the construction of brain states. The methodological question that arises is that of generating a descriptive approach relating functional neuroimaging data to whole brain dynamics. Recent attempts to address this question have adopted two approaches. The first employs a BOLD, data-driven, computational method that leverages the method of *recurrence structure analysis* (RSA), a mathematical procedure derived from Poincare's recurrence theorem [41]. This "recurrent" behavior can be described by a *recurrence plot method* (RP), which allows a matrix-based visualization of recurrent states. The second approach posits the governance of RSN dynamics by a ground state global attractor. This global ground state is mathematically described as a stable stationary solution representing a point of maximal stability in a landscape of stationary points (nodes) that information flows toward or away from [42]. This theoretical framework has been shown to successfully account for the highly structured dynamics arising from spontaneous brain activity in RSNs [43].

6. Conclusion and future directions

Building on Bloch and Purcell's method for detecting the nuclear magnetic resonance phenomenon, clinical applications have evolved at virtually all stages along the MRI procedural pipeline. Long intervals for data acquisition that plagued early clinical use have been substantially lessened; algorithms for preprocessing with co-registration and denoising have become routine; machine learning for tissue-specific fingerprinting and feature extraction has been introduced, and functional methods for cardiac and brain diagnosis are reliably and regularly used. Future directions will see the roles of adjunct computational resources continue to grow. MRI has traditionally been a procedure for structural tissue determinations, and the assessing of structural differences between normal and trauma or disease states has typically been performed by clinicians. Aiding them will be new algorithms and enhanced computational power for improved feature extraction and pattern recognition capabilities.

Clinical diagnoses will increasingly rely on dynamic and physiological parameters associated with functional performance.

In the nervous system, the drive to consolidate improved temporal resolution with the current abilities for high spatial resolution, for instance, will seek to enlist methods successfully used for high spatial resolution in novel ways that match neuronal activity timescales, such as the interleaving of K-space data coupled with theoretical models that enable direct neural activity monitoring. Noninvasive techniques will also introduce perturbation studies to monitor how these influence brain dynamics. Together, these and other innovations will amplify the already leading clinical role of MRI-based applications.

Author details

Denis Larrivee[1,2]

1 Mind and Brain Institute, University of Navarra Medical School, Spain

2 Loyola University Chicago, USA

*Address all correspondence to: sallar1@aol.com

References

[1] Smith FW, Hutchison JM, Mallard JR, et al. Oesophageal carcinoma demonstrated by whole-body nuclear magnetic resonance imaging. British Medical Journal (Clinical Research Edition). 1981;**282**(6263):510-512

[2] Bloch F, Hansen WW, Packard ME. Nuclear induction. Physics Review. 1946;**69**:127

[3] Purcell EM, Torrey HC, Pound RV. Resonance absorption by nuclear magnetic moments in a solid. Physics Review. 1946;**69**:37-38

[4] Grover VPB, Tognarelli JM, Crossey MME, et al. Magnetic resonance imaging: Principles and techniques: Lessons for clinicians. Journal of Clinical and Experimental Hepatology. 2015;**5**(3):246-255

[5] Moratal D, Vallés-Luch A, Martí-Bonmatí L, Brummer M. k-space tutorial: An MRI educational tool for a better understanding of k-space. Biomedical Imaging Intervention Journal. 2008;**4**(1):e15. DOI: 10.2349/biij.4.1.e15

[6] Mezrich R. A perspective on K space. Radiology. 1995;**195**(2):297-315

[7] Sýkora S. K space formulation of MRI. In: Sykora S, editor. Stan's Library. Vol. Volume I. Castano Primo, Italy: Permalink; 2005

[8] Deshmane A, Eng M, Gulani V, et al. Parallel MR imaging. Journal of Magnetic Resonance Imaging. 2012;**36**(1):55-72. DOI: 10.1002/jmri.23639

[9] Gomez A, Molina-Romera M, Buonincontri G, et al. Designing contrasts for rapid, simultaneous parameter quantification and flow visualization with quantitative transient-state imaging. Journal of Clinical and Experimental Hepatology. 2015;**5**(3):246-255

[10] Yang J, Gohel S, Vachha B. Current methods and new directions in resting state fMRI. Clinical Imaging. 2020;**65**:47-53. DOI: 10.1016/j.clinimag.2020.04.004

[11] Vadmal V, Junno G, Badye C, et al. MRI image analysis methods and applications. Neuro-Oncology Advances. 2020;**2**(1):1-13

[12] Gordon Y, Partovi S, Müller-Eschner M, et al. Dynamic contrast-enhanced magnetic resonance imaging: Fundamentals and application to the evaluation of the peripheral perfusion. Cardiovascular Diagnostic Therapy. 2014;**4**(2):147-164. DOI: 10.3978/j.issn.2223-3652.2014.03.01

[13] Bandettini P. The spatial, temporal, and interpretive limits of functional MRI. In: Davis K, Charney D, Coyle JT, Nemeroff C, editors. Neuropsychopharmacology: The Fifth Generation of Progress. Philadelphia: Lippincott, Williams, and Wilkins; 2002

[14] Hamilton J, Franson D, Seiberlich N. Recent advances in parallel imaging for MRI. Progress in Nuclear Magnetic Resonance Spectroscopy. 2017;**101**:71-95. DOI: 10.1016/j.pnmrs.2017.04.002

[15] Calogero C. Recent advances in parallel imaging for MRI: WAVE-CAIPI technique. Journal of Advanced Health Care. 2022;**4**(1):23-26

[16] Khalila M, Ayada H, Adiba A. Performance evaluation of feature extraction techniques in MR-brain image

classification system. Procedia Computer Science. 2018;**127**:218-225

[17] Fayaz M, Torokeldiev N, Turdumamatov S, et al. An efficient methodology for brain MRI classification based on DWT and convolutional neural network. Sensors. 2021;**21**:7480. DOI: 10.3390/s21227480

[18] Ma D, Gulani V, Seiberlich N, et al. Magnctic rcsonancc fingerprinting. Nature. 2013;**495**:187-192

[19] Zhao B, Haldar JP, Setsompop K, Wald LL. Optimal experiment design for magnetic resonance fingerprinting. In: 2016 38th Annual International Conference of the IEEE Engineering in Medicine and Biology Society (EMBC). Lake Buena Vista, FL. pp. 453-456. DOI: 10.1109

[20] Liao C, Bilzic B, Manhard MK, et al. 3D MR fingerprinting with accelerated stack-of-spirals and hybrid sliding-window and GRAPPA reconstruction. NeuroImage. 2017;**162**:13-22. DOI: 10.1016/j.neuroimage.2017.08.030

[21] Marty B, Carlier PG. Physiological and pathological skeletal muscle T1 changes quantified using a fast inversion-recovery radial NMR imaging sequence. Science Reports. 2019;**9**:6852. DOI: 10.1038/s41598-019-43398-x

[22] Buonincontri G, Sawiak S. Three-dimensional MR fingerprinting with simultaneous B1 estimation. Magnetic Resonance Medicine. 2015;**2015**:1-9

[23] Cao X et al. A model-based velocity mapping of blood flow using MR fingerprinting. Proceedings of the International Society for Magnetic Resonance in Medicine. 2017;**25**:0941

[24] Loued-Khenissi L, Doll O, Preuschoff K. An overview of functional magnetic resonance imaging techniques for organizational research. Organizational Research Methods. 2019;**22**(1):17-45

[25] Yacoub E, Van De Moortele PF, Shmuel A, et al. Signal and noise characteristics of Hahn SE and GE BOLD fMRI at 7 T in humans. NeuroImage. 2005;**2005**(24):738-750. DOI: 10.1016/j.neuroimage

[26] Pohmann R, Speck O, Scheffler K. 2016. Signal-to-noise ratio and MR tissue parameters in human brain imaging at 3, 7, and 9.4 Tesla using current receive coil arrays. Magnetic Resonance Medicine. 2016;**75**:801-809. DOI: 10.1002/mrm.25677

[27] Branco P, Seixas D, Castro SL. Temporal reliability of ultra-high field resting- state MRI for single-subject sensorimotor and language mapping. NeuroImage. 2018;**168**:499-508. DOI: 10.1016/j.neuroimage.2016.11.029

[28] Raimondo L, Icaro AF, Jurjen HO, et al. Advances in resting state fMRI acquisitions for functional connectomics. NeuroImage. 2021;**243**:118503

[29] Van de Moortele PF, Auerbach EJ, Olman C, et al. T1 weighted brain images at 7 Tesla unbiased for proton density, T2* contrast and RF coil receive B1 sensitivity with simultaneous vessel visualization. NeuroImage. 2009;**46**:432-446. DOI: 10.1016/j.neuroimage.2009.02.009

[30] Fleury M, Figueiredo P, Vourvopoulos A, and Lécuyer A. Two is better? Combining EEG and fMRI for BCI and Neurofeedback: A systematic review. 2023. hal-04038069

[31] Toi PT, Jang JH, Kyeong SM, et al. In vivo direct imaging of neuronal activity at high temporospatial resolution. Science. 2022;**378**(6616): 160-168. DOI: 10.1126/science.abh43

[32] Biswal B, Yetkin FZ, Haughton VM, Hyde JS. Functional connectivity in the motor cortex of resting human brain using echo-planar MRI. Magnetic Resonance Medicine. 1995;**34**(4): 537-541. DOI: 10.1002/mrm.1910340409

[33] Damoiseaux SA, Rombouts RB, Barkhof F, Beckman CF. Consistent resting-state networks across healthy subjects. Proceedings of the National Academy of Sciences. 2006;**103**(37):13848-13853. DOI: 10.1073

[34] Ogawa S, Tank DW, Menon R, et al. Intrinsic signal changes accompanying sensory stimulation: Functional brain mapping with magnetic resonance imaging. Proceedings of the National Academy of Science USA. 1992;**89**:5951-5955

[35] Yeo BTT, Krienen FM, Sepulcre J, et al. The organization of the human cerebral cortex estimated by intrinsic functional connectivity. Journal of Neurophysiology. 2011;**106**:1125-1165. DOI: 10.1152/jn.00338.2011

[36] Smitha KA, Akhil RK, Arun KM, et al. Resting state fMRI: A review on methods in resting state connectivity analysis and resting state networks. The Neuroradiology Journal. 2017;**30**(4):305-317. DOI: 10.1177/1971400917697342

[37] Corbetta M, Siegel JS, Schulman GL. On the low dimensionality of behavioral deficits and alterations of brain network connectivity after focal injury. Cortex. 2018;**107**:229-237

[38] Lerman-Sinkoff DB, Barch DM. Network community structure alterations in adult schizophrenia: Identification and localization of alterations. Neuroimage Clinic. 2016;**10**:96-106. DOI: 10.1016/j.nicl.2015.11.011

[39] Bullmore ET, Sporns O. Complex brain networks: Graph theoretical analysis of structural and functional systems. Nature Review Neuroscience. 2009;**10**:186-198. DOI: 10.1038/nrn2575

[40] Lee WH, Frangou S. Linking functional connectivity and dynamic properties of resting-state networks. Scientific Reports. 2017;**7**:16610. DOI: 10.1038/s41598-017-16789-1

[41] Beim Graben P, Jimenez-Marin A, Diez I, Cortes JM, et al. Metastable resting state brain dynamics. Frontiers in Computational Neuroscience. 2019;**13**:62. DOI: 10.3389/fncom.2019.00062

[42] Carvalho A, Langa J, Robinson J. Attractors for Infinite-Dimensional Non-autonomous Dynamical Systems. New York: Springer; 2012

[43] Gonzalez L, Panda R, Ponce-Alvarez A, et al. Loss of consciousness reduces the stability of brain hubs and the heterogeneity of brain dynamics. Communications Biology. 2021;**4**(1):34489535

Section 2

Dynamic MRI in Cardiovascular Diagnosis

Chapter 2

State of the Art and New Advances: Cardiac MRI

Hunter Frederiksen, Corina Iorgoveanu and Mahi L. Ashwath

Abstract

Cardiac Magnetic Resonance Imaging (CMR) is an advanced imaging modality for better assessment of cardiac structure, function and tissue characterization. This is an essential imaging modality when indicated for assessment of a variety of cardiomyopathies, cardiac ischemia, myocardial viability, arrhythmias, cardiac masses, congenital heart disease, shunts, acute and constrictive pericardial diseases among others. CMR is sometimes referred to as the non-invasive biopsy given the significant information it provides. This chapter discusses the current state of the art of CMR with discussion about the indications, common sequences used, and the role of CMR in evaluation of ischemic and non-ischemic cardiac disease. This chapter also discusses new advances and the future of the field of CMR.

Keywords: CMR, ischemic cardiomyopathy, non-ischemic cardiomyopathy, cardiac masses, pericardial disease, arrhythmias, advances in CMR

1. Introduction

Imaging the heart using magnetic resonance imaging (MRI) started for diagnostic utilization in the 1980s and has since contributed to significant advances in the fields of adult and pediatric cardiology and cardiothoracic surgery. Cardiac MRI (CMR) provides precise visualization of myocardial structure, function, perfusion, viability, and tissue characterization offering a comprehensive evaluation that remains unparalleled by any other imaging technique. Compared to other cardiac imaging modalities such as transthoracic echocardiogram (TTE), transesophageal echocardiogram (TEE), cardiac catheterization, or cardiac computed tomographic angiography (CTA), CMR has the advantages of reliable, high quality imaging with advanced tissue characterization which is not limited by body habitus, does not have radiation, is noninvasive, and has been shown to be sufficient for disease characterization and subsequent treatment strategies [1] aiding in tailoring specific treatment options and enhancing patient outcomes. Over the years, CMR with a continuing addition of several new techniques, has proven to be critically important for cardiovascular disease characterization and subsequent management and outcomes. We discuss the indications for CMR, common CMR scanning sequences, current state of the art of CMR followed by advances in CMR.

2. Indications for CMR

CMR should be considered as part of the diagnostic imaging in patients with

- Acute and chronic coronary artery disease
- Evaluation of ischemia in patients with chest pain
- Non ischemic cardiomyopathy, especially when the etiology of non-ischemic cardiomyopathy is unclear, or for prognosis in patients after etiology of non-ischemic cardiomyopathy is identified
- Valvular heart disease
- Cardiac masses
- Pericardial disease
- Cardiac arrhythmias including brady arrhythmias, complete heart block, ventricular arrhythmias, and sudden cardiac death
- Congenital heart disease (CHD)—simple CHD like atrial septal defects or ventricular septal defects or complex CHD like Tetralogy of Fallot, transposition of great arteries, truncus arteriosus and single ventricle physiology for diagnosis and for serial follow up
- Aortic diseases including coarctation, aneurysm, dissection, and vasculitis
- Anomalous coronaries or anomalous pulmonary veins

3. Scanning protocol and sequences

A regular CMR uses cine images for function and morphology followed by delayed enhancement (DE) images after administration of contrast for scar evaluation. While the scan as described provides significant information, additional information can be obtained, using additional sequences as desired. The study and the sequences are usually tailored for the indication to meet the needs appropriately. Commonly used sequences in CMR scanning include:

1. Steady state Free Precession (SSFP) or cine imaging provides high quality still or moving images for evaluation of structure and function. Image acquisition must be coupled to an EKG to gather adequate data over successive heartbeats. The lack of limitations of body habitus along with the superior contrast resolution and improved differentiation between blood pool and muscle are the advantages with CMR (Video 1).

2. DE imaging for late gadolinium enhancement (LGE) is performed a few minutes after injecting Gadolinium for evaluation of scar or infiltration using phase contrast inversion recovery or PSIR sequences (**Figure 1**). DE Images are obtained at

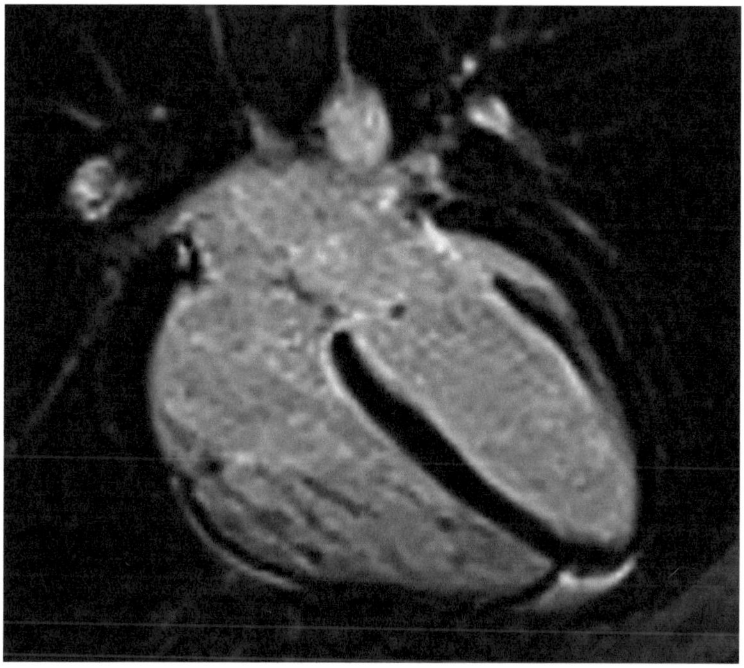

Figure 1.
Normal DE imaging with myocardium appearing uniformly black.

a set time point post-contrast injection to evaluate how the contrast distributes into the extracellular space. LGE patterns on delayed enhancement imaging assist in the differentiation of ischemic and nonischemic cardiomyopathies. LGE in nonischemic cardiomyopathy is present in a noncoronary distribution and can have diffuse myocardial, mid myocardial or epicardial enhancement. Ischemic cardiomyopathy always has subendocardial involvement due to coronary blood flow pattern. Quantifying LGE and thereby assessing scar burden can provide prognostic and outcomes information. Studies have showed that presence of LGE in cardiomyopathy patients was associated with an increased risk of all-cause mortality, hospitalization for heart failure, and sudden cardiac death (SCD) [2].

3. Real time cine sequences are used in patients with arrhythmias for structure and function or routinely in patients being evaluated for constrictive pericarditis and ventricular interdependence and have a more continuous acquisition (Video 2)

4. T1 and T2 mapping and parametric imaging sequences for tissue characterization are excellent for assessing diffuse and localized myocardial inflammation, infiltration, edema, intracellular and extracellular volume, and fibrosis (**Figure 2**). Extracellular volume (ECV) is measured by analyzing T1 values pre- and post-contrast and has been found useful in identifying edema or fibrosis specific to cardiac diseases [3]. T1, T2 and ECV evaluation provides prognostic information in addition to aiding in the diagnosis.

5. T2* sequences for myocardial iron content can assist in the evaluation of myocardial iron content in diseases characterized by iron deposition.

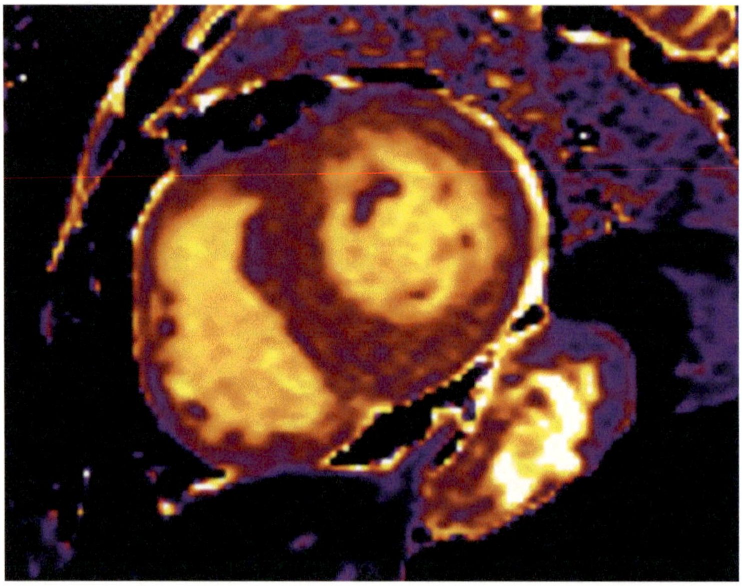

Figure 2.
T1 mapping sequence.

6. Perfusion CMR is a technique that uses contrast dynamics to visualize saturations of blood flow into the myocardium. Perfusion imaging is used for assessment of perfusion of myocardium and cardiac masses when present (Video 3).

7. Phase contrast velocity encoded sequences or flow sequences for hemodynamic assessment for assessment of flows, peak velocity, gradients and volumes.

8. Contrast-enhanced CMR angiography (MRA) for assessment of vascular structures. 3-Dimensional (3D) visualization and accurate assessment can be performed for aneurysms, dissections, vasculitis, or congenital heart disease (Video 4).

4. Current state of the art of CMR

CMR has extensive role in the evaluation of various ischemic and non-ischemic etiologies. A few of the common pathologies are discussed below.

4.1 Evaluation of ischemic heart disease

Coronary artery disease (CAD) is the leading cause of death in the United States. One person dies every 33 seconds from cardiovascular disease in the United States [4]. CMR has unique value in the evaluation of acute and chronic ischemic heart disease and in patients presenting with chest pain for the evaluation of ischemia.

4.1.1 Acute ischemic heart disease and CMR

CMR provides many insights in the evaluation of patients presenting with acute MI. While TTE is easily accessible, CMR is superior to TTE in the evaluation wall motion abnormalities and LV ejection fraction (EF) with high quality imaging in cine sequences. CMR provides additional information about edema and the area at risk of infarction which can be evaluated by T1, T2 mapping and assessment of ECV. Resting myocardial perfusion imaging in patients presenting with chest pain can show areas of decreased resting myocardial perfusion, denoting significant coronary stenosis (greater than 80% stenosis) in the coronary arteries supplying those territories [5] (Video 5). Early gadolinium imaging shows areas of thrombus (**Figure 3**) and microvascular obstruction (**Figure 4**). Microvascular obstruction signifies areas with extensive ischemia with associated capillary cell death in addition to myocardial cell death. Presence of microvascular ischemia portends a worse prognosis compared to patients who do not have microvascular ischemia [6] LGE on DE imaging

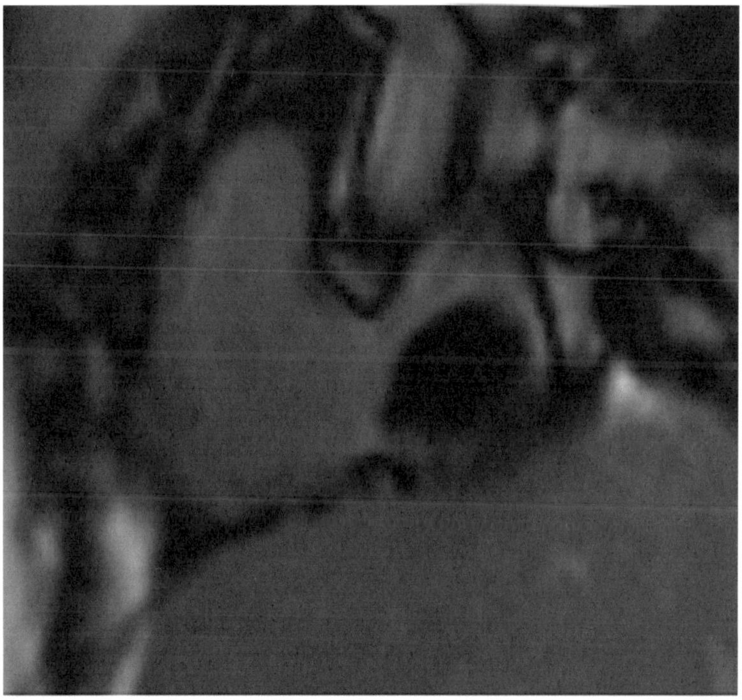

Figure 3.
Early gadolinium imaging with a right atrial thrombus as hypointense lesion.

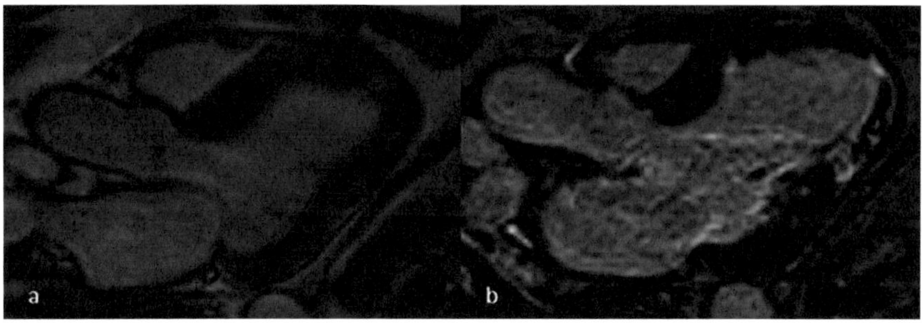

Figure 4.
Cine image (a) and DE imaging (b) in acute MI showing a significant dark zone of microvascular obstruction embedded within the infarcted area in the mid to apical inferolateral wall.

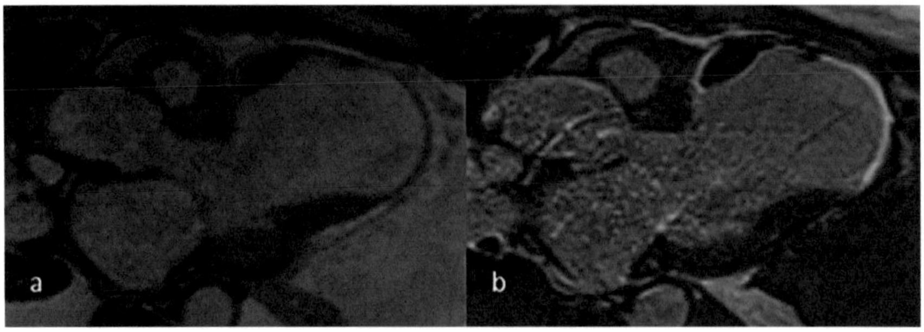

Figure 5.
Cine image (a) and DE imaging (b) in MI showing bright scar tissue in LAD territory, signifying lack of viable myocardium with superimposed thrombus in black.

shows areas of myocardial scar [7] (**Figure 5**). Ischemic scar always involves the sub endocardium as shown on pathology studies. Studies have shown that myocardium with less than 50% involvement of the myocardial thickness with scar have improvement in function with revascularization, suggestive of viable myocardium, while segments with more than 50% wall thickness involvement with scar do not have functional recovery [7]. Assessment of viable myocardium can have value in deciding revascularization strategies. CMR also plays an important role in the evaluation of complications of acute MI such as pseudoaneurysm (Video 6), thrombus, rupture of the septum, myocardial free wall rupture or papillary muscle rupture. Above findings, especially LV EF, microvascular obstruction and degree of scar have been shown to have prognostic valve.

4.1.2 Chronic ischemic heart disease and CMR

In patients with chronic CAD, CMR provides information about EF with cine imaging, thrombus evaluation with cine, early gadolinium enhancement, LGE imaging as described in the above section along with the detection and quantification of scar. Despite its widespread availability, TTE can be diagnostically limited in evaluation of intracardiac thrombus. Studies comparing TTE, TEE and CMR have clearly demonstrated the superiority of CMR in diagnosing thrombi [8]. CMR imaging provides tissue characterization of thrombus and can identify structural risk factors for LV thrombus such as infarct size/distribution and contractile dysfunction [9]. Presence of scar in myocardial infarcts can be most accurately detected by CMR compared to any other imaging study [10]. Transmural scar shows non-viable myocardium and identifies patients who are less likely to improve function [11]. Studies in patients with non-Q wave MI and unstable angina demonstrated the importance of subendocardial scar detected in CMR and its prognostic value [12]. Other studies have shown how these subendocardial scars can be easily missed on single-photon emission computed tomography (SPECT) imaging. Above findings, especially LV EF, and degree of scar have been shown to have prognostic valve.

4.1.3 Evaluation of ischemia in patients with chest pain and CMR

CMR provides valuable information in the evaluation of chest pain or ischemia with stress testing. Perfusion CMR, a technique that uses contrast dynamics to visualize saturations of blood flow into the myocardium is used in stress perfusion CMR. In stress CMR, Gadolinium based contrast agent is paired with a vasodilator such as adenosine or Regadenoson and images are obtained continuously over several cardiac cycles to visualize the myocardial uptake and fade-out of contrast. In healthy myocardium, the contrast distributes homogenously. Defects in perfusion are typically detected as areas of low contrast resulting in minimal signal and therefore representing hypoperfusion and must last for four or more consecutive cardiac cycles [13]. Studies such as CE MARC showed the non-inferiority of Stress CMR compared to SPECT [14]. The GadaCad trial which compared Stress CMR to invasive coronary angiography or coronary CTA as the reference standard showed that stress CMR had sensitivities of 79% and 87% and specificities of 87% and 73% for single- and multi-vessel CAD, respectively. Studies such as SPINS showed the prognostic value of Stress CMR with patients with normal Stress CMR—patients with normal myocardial perfusion and normal LGE have 99.3% event free survival for a median 5.5 years [15].

When compared to SPECT, stress CMR has several technical advantages. CMR has a larger field of view, superior spatial resolution, and better tissue differentiation. It is not limited by attenuation artifacts or contamination of the myocardium by other signal sources such as gut uptake as can be the case with SPECT. Stress CMR can also identify subendocardial ischemia, making it less susceptible to balanced ischemia than SPECT, where multivessel ischemia may be present but falsely appear normal on perfusion images [16]. Additionally, stress CMR does not expose patients to ionizing radiation, making it advantageous for younger patients and those who require multiple scans over time.

4.2 Evaluation of non-ischemic heart disease (NICM)

The present classification system for cardiomyopathies, established by the American Heart Association distinguishes between primary ones that solely impact the heart and secondary ones that are part of a larger systemic disease affecting multiple organs. CMR has a distinct advantage in evaluation of these cardiomyopathies by providing insights into tissue composition and characteristics beyond structural imaging.

4.2.1 Primary cardiomyopathies

4.2.1.1 Hypertrophic cardiomyopathy (HCM)

HCM is a genetic cardiomyopathy, characterized by myocardial hypertrophy and disarray with an estimated prevalence of 1 in 500. CMR excels in identifying location and degree of hypertrophy, accurate maximal wall thickness, systolic anterior motion of the mitral valve and LV outflow tract obstruction, LV crypts, aneurysms and morphological variations involving the mitral valve apparatus and papillary muscles (Video 7). The classic scar pattern in HCM involves LGE at right ventricular (RV) insertion points [17] (**Figure 6**). A comprehensive multicenter study involving nearly 1300 patients diagnosed with HCM revealed that the extent of LGE can effectively identify individuals who are at an elevated risk of sudden death who would need to be considered for implantable cardioverter-defibrillator (ICD) placement. Extensive LGE, encompassing 15% or more of the LV mass, indicates a twofold higher risk of sudden death compared to the absence of LGE [18].

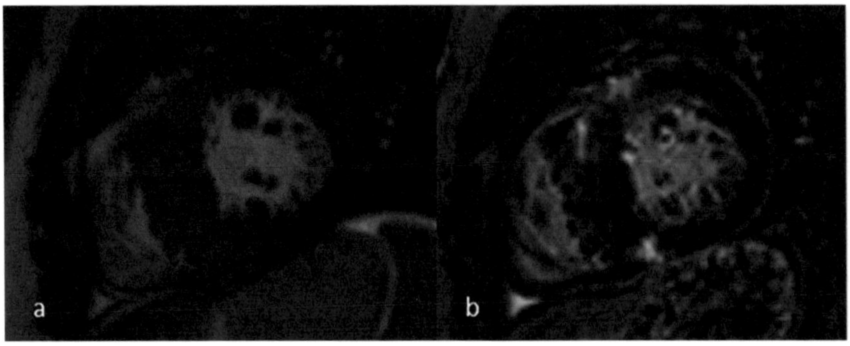

Figure 6.
Short axis cine (a) and DE (b) showing septal hypertrophy with LGE at RV insertion points in HCM.

4.2.1.2 Arrhythmogenic right ventricular cardiomyopathy (ARVC)

ARVC, the most prominent form of heritable arrhythmogenic cardiomyopathy (ACM), is a genetic disorder that is characterized by the loss of myocytes and the replacement of myocardial tissue with fibrofatty deposits, primarily affecting the RV. ARVC is associated with the occurrence of ventricular arrhythmias and an elevated risk of SCD and heart failure. Given the limitations of TTE in the visualization of the RV, CMR is the preferred diagnostic test for this lethal cardiomyopathy. CMR offers a comprehensive assessment of RV for enlargement of the RV outflow tract, dilation of the RV, fibrofatty replacement of the myocardium, as well as global or regional systolic dysfunction (Video 8). According to the 2010 Task Force Criteria, qualitative CMR identification of increased RV end-diastolic volumes, RV akinesia, dyskinesia, or dyssynchronous RV contraction is necessary to fulfill major or minor diagnostic criteria.

In the coming years, the analysis of tissue deformation and strain using CMR holds the potential to offer valuable diagnostic and prognostic insights. Strain imaging has shown promise in distinguishing individuals with ARVC and borderline ARVC from healthy volunteers, as well as differentiating it from other conditions like right ventricular outflow-tract ventricular tachycardia (RVOT-ventricular tachycardia) and Brugada syndrome. Impaired strain in both the LV and RV is indicative of ARVC. Emerging techniques, such as water and fat separation and high-resolution 3D LGE imaging hold potential for enhancing the identification of ARVC [19].

4.2.1.3 Left ventricular non-compaction (LVNC)

LVNC refers to a structural configuration of the LV wall that is distinguished by prominent trabeculae within the LV, a thin layer of compacted myocardium, and deep recesses between the trabeculae. CMR cine images offer superior contrast resolution and improved differentiation between blood and muscle, enabling clearer visualization of ventricular trabeculation (**Figure 7**). Various CMR criteria have been proposed, with the criterion introduced by Petersen et al. being the most utilized. According to this criterion, a ratio of trabecular to compact myocardial thicknesses greater than 2.3 at end-diastole in long-axis views is consistent with noncompaction cardiomyopathy [20]. With the help of LGE in LVNC, regions of LGE in the

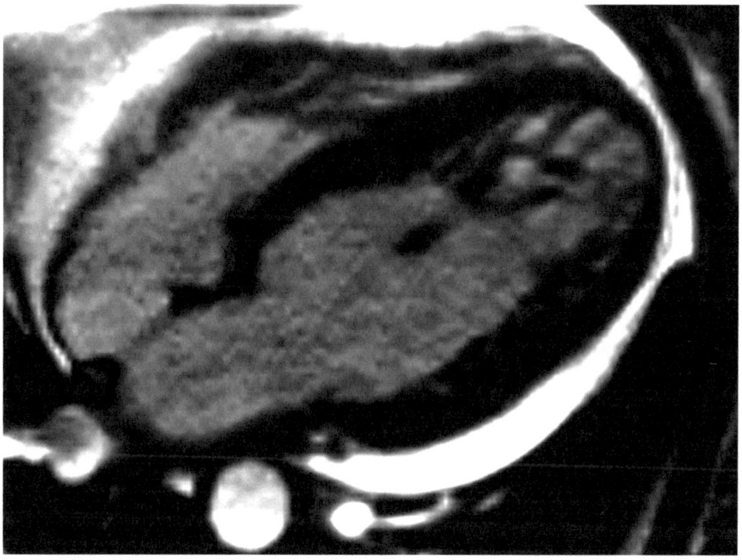

Figure 7.
Four chamber cine images with non-compacted myocardium in the mid to apical segments.

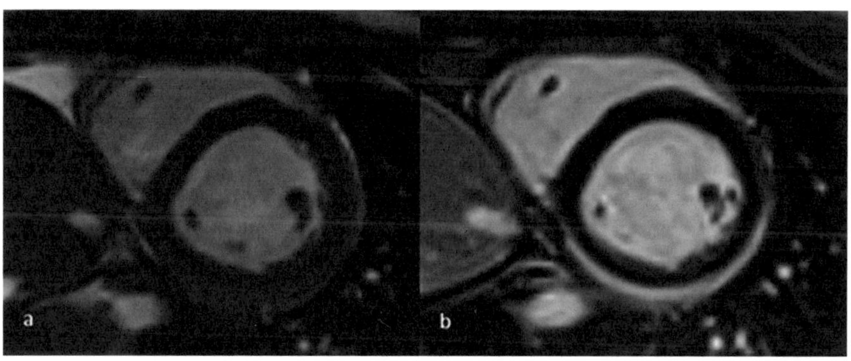

Figure 8.
Short axis cine (a) and DE (b) imaging showing the inferolateral epicardial scar in myocarditis.

trabecular and subendocardial layers can be observed, indicating the presence of subendocardial and trabecular fibrosis as well as fibroelastosis. These fibrotic areas serve as the substrate for potentially life-threatening arrhythmias, which are the primary cause of sudden death in affected patients [21].

4.2.1.4 Myocarditis

Myocarditis is an inflammatory condition of the myocardium, which can arise due to various causes, including a broad spectrum of infectious and noninfectious etiologies [22]. CMR detects several cardinal features of myocarditis such as inflammation, edema, necrosis, and contractile dysfunction (**Figure 6**) [23]. Cine images assist with assessment of wall motion abnormalities, T1 and T2 mapping with assessment for ECV and myocardial edema and DE imaging with assessment for focal scars. DE is typically observed in a mid-myocardial or sub-epicardial pattern primarily affecting the basal to mid inferolateral and inferior segments [24] (**Figure 8**). The Lake Louise Criteria aid in the decision making by using CMR to detect myocarditis with high specificity and positive predictive value [3].

4.2.2 Secondary cardiomyopathies

4.2.2.1 Cardiac amyloidosis

Amyloidosis is a rare medical condition that arises due to the accumulation of insoluble proteinaceous material in the extracellular matrix. The likelihood of amyloidosis affecting the heart varies depending on the specific type, with primary/AL type having the highest incidence of cardiac involvement, affecting up to 50% of patients, followed by familial/ATTR type affecting 10–50% of patients, while the incidence is less than 5% for secondary/AA type [25]. CMR can detect key features of cardiac amyloid and can serve to rule in or rule out a diagnosis of cardiac amyloidosis [26]. The presence of the abnormal protein in the myocardium affects its T1 relaxation, making it challenging to null the myocardium and resulting in increased T1 values, which can be quantified using mapping techniques. ECV calculates the extracellular expansion due to amyloid and represents the closest, non-invasive quantification of cardiac amyloid burden. DE imaging shows a global subendocardial or transmural patchy enhancement (**Figure 9**). The presence and the degree of enhancement have been shown to have prognostic value in addition to the prognostic value provided by T1 and ECV values [27–29].

4.2.2.2 Sarcoidosis

Sarcoidosis is a destructive granulomatous disease of the myocardium, which can lead to several cardiac pathologies including heart failure, heart blocks, ventricular arrythmias, and SCD. Diagnosing cardiac sarcoidosis is a challenge as symptoms often mimic other cardiac conditions. Autopsy studies have shown that isolated cardiac sarcoidosis can occur, and cardiac arrhythmias can be the first presentation [29]. Currently, the best imaging modalities for detecting sarcoid inflammation are cardiac positron emission tomography (CPET) and CMR [30]. CPET is useful for detecting active areas of inflammation and can provide good insight into disease burden. CMR on the other hand can show active areas of inflammation using T1 and

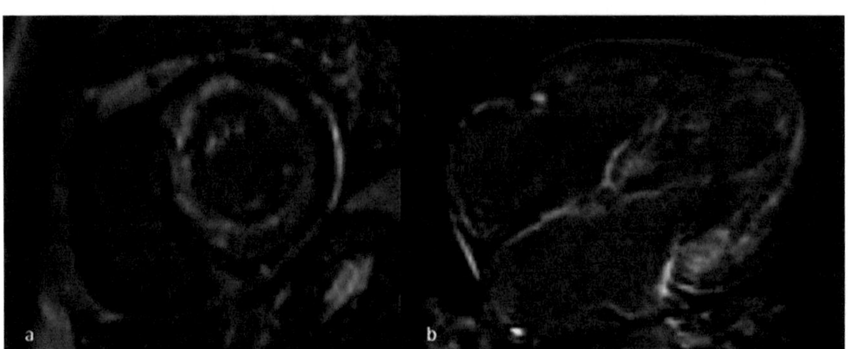

Figure 9.
Global subendocardial (a) and diffuse (b) enhancement in amyloidosis.

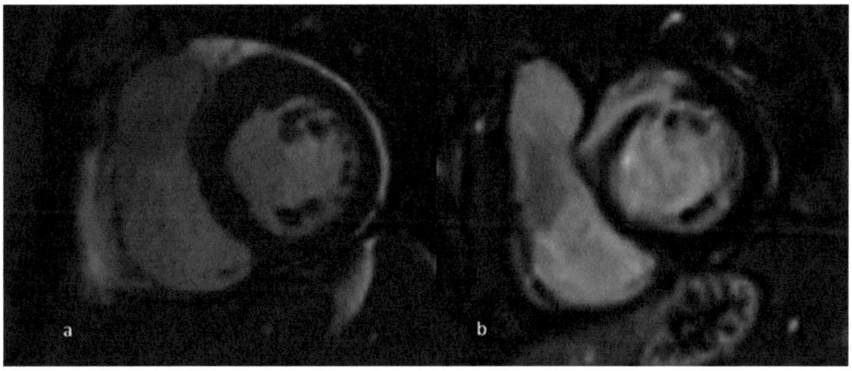

Figure 10.
Short axis cine (a) and DE (b) imaging showing epicardial and septal scar in sarcoidosis.

T2 mapping in addition to detecting areas of involved myocardium and scar tissue left over from active disease with DE imaging (**Figure 10**). The societal recommendation for imaging cardiac sarcoidosis involves obtaining cine, LGE, resting perfusion and T2-weighted sequences [31]. Regional wall motion abnormalities with cine imaging, focal perfusion abnormalities during perfusion imaging, signs of inflammation and edema during the acute phase of the disease on T1-weighted images [25], epicardial, midmyocardial DE and RV involvement with wall motion abnormalities and scarring have all been reported. Scar tissue serves as the epicenter for developing arrythmias. CMR locates and quantifies scar tissue burden and can aid in predicting risk for fatal arrythmias and patients that need treatment with an ICD [32].

4.2.2.3 Fabry cardiomyopathy

Fabry disease (FD) is a lysosomal storage disorder that presents with a range of cardiac manifestations such as ventricular hypertrophy and fibrosis, valve thickening or regurgitation, heart failure, angina, dysrhythmias, cardiac conduction abnormalities, and SCD [33]. CMR has contributed significantly to our understanding of the underlying processes that lead to inflammation and fibrosis as a response to the accumulation of glycosphingolipids [34]. Earlier in the disease when the characteristic feature is fatty changes, decrease in native T1 time occurs [35]. This finding has the potential to identify individuals with early cardiac involvement and has been demonstrated to be predictive of disease progression [34]. As the disease progresses, the fatty changes are replaced with fibrosis, which leads to increase in T1 values along with patchy enhancement which is typically seen in the basal inferolateral wall [33] (**Figure 11**). These changes can occur concurrently with fatty changes in the septum and fibrosis in the inferolateral wall with rate of disease progression varying in different segments. These changes can also happen prior to the detection of LV hypertrophy, leading to early diagnosis.

4.2.2.4 Endomyocardial fibrosis (EMF)

EMF is a type of restrictive cardiomyopathy, and although no exact cause has been fully understood, various factors have been described that contribute to an inflammatory response, leading to damage in the endomyocardial layers and the subsequent formation of fibrosis [36]. On CMR cine images shows apical

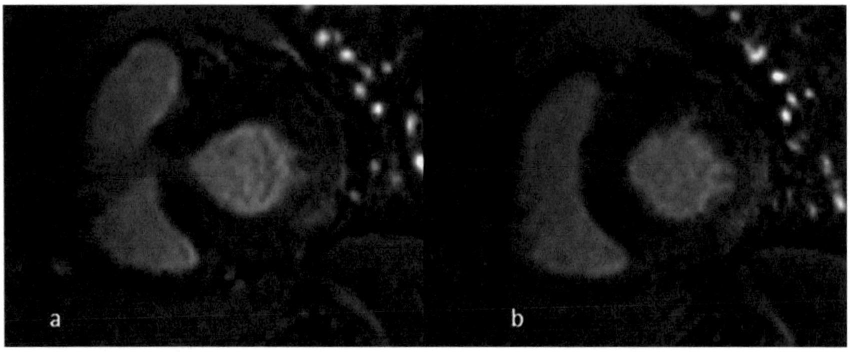

Figure 11.
Short axis basal (a) and mid-level (b) DE imaging showing inferolateral patchy enhancement in Fabry cardiomyopathy.

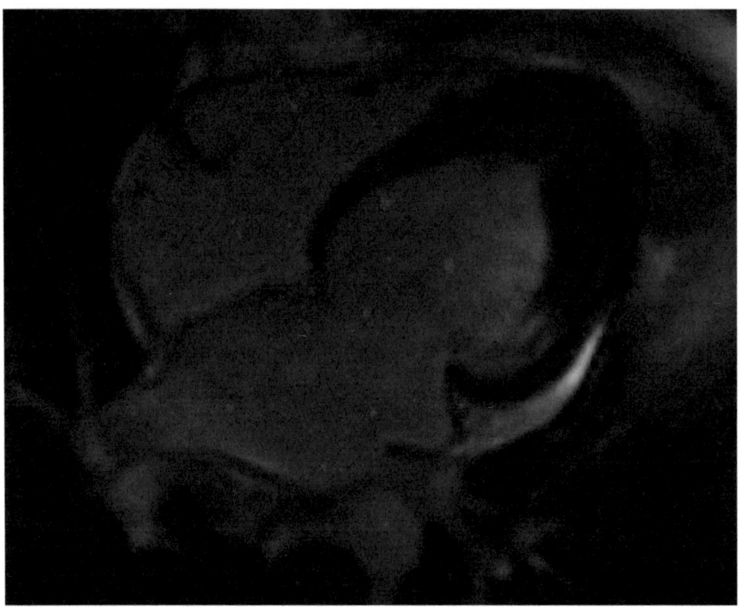

Figure 12.
Cine imaging in endomyocardial fibrosis showing apical hypertrophy.

hypertrophic pattern, (**Figure 12**) however LGE serves as a dependable noninvasive approach for diagnosing EMF. The characteristic DE pattern observed in EMF is subendocardial, not limited to a specific coronary distribution with overlying thrombus. It primarily affects the apical walls of the LV and may extend continuously to the inflow tract. At the ventricular apex, a distinct imaging feature known as a "double V" sign can be observed. This sign exhibits a three-layered appearance comprising normal myocardium, enhanced endomyocardium and a layer of thrombus (**Figure 13**). CMR findings also have prognostic value. An increased deposition of apical fibrous tissue, indexed to body surface area (BSA) (>19 mL/m^2), has been directly associated with worse New York Heart Association (NYHA) functional class and elevated mortality rates [37].

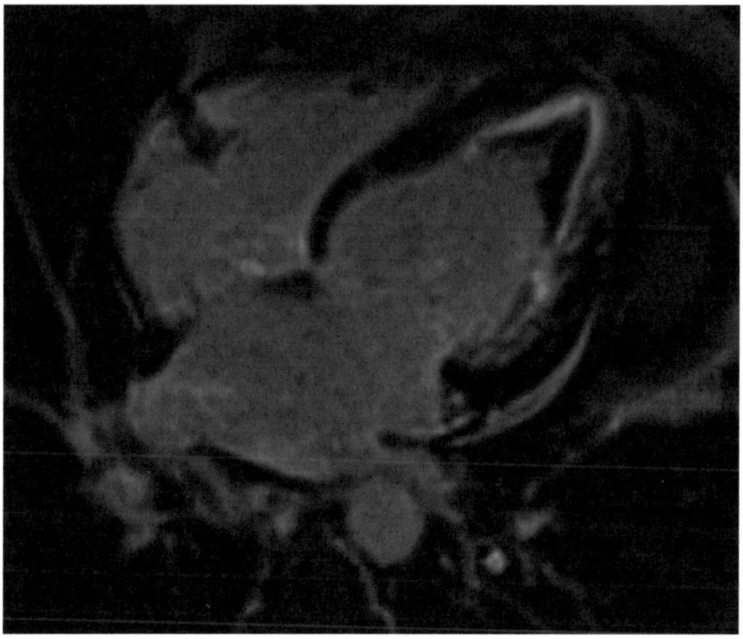

Figure 13.
DE imaging in endomyocardial fibrosis showing apical to mid ventricular scar with superimposed thrombus.

4.3 Valvular heart disease

Over the last two decades CMR has emerged as a non-invasive and radiation-free alternative that can be used in individuals with valvular heart disease. CMR can provide images of valve anatomy and enables the quantitative evaluation of stenosis and regurgitation. Cine imaging assists with assessment the valvular structures in motion along with visualization of flows. Phase-contrast velocity encoded sequences help with quantification of peak velocities and regurgitant fractions. CMR can also detect the consequences of valvular lesions, such as changes in systolic function and the effects of ventricular volume or pressure overload [38]. Time-resolved 3D phase-contrast MRI, also known as 4D flow MRI, is a newer sequence, that possesses impressive capabilities in measuring blood flow velocities within a volume, noninvasively and in vivo, across the three primary directions, enabling the dynamic assessment of blood flow in both the heart and major vessels [38].

4.4 Cardiac masses

Either of primary or secondary origin, cardiac masses can have various tissue compositions such as myxomas, rhabdomyomas, fibromas, angiosarcomas, and metastasis from extra-cardiac cancers. The characterization of cardiac masses is based on size, location, interaction with surrounding structures and mobility [39]. The first level of diagnostics remains to be an TTE as it is widely available, convenient, and of relatively minimal cost but has its own limitations. CMR can provide a multiplanar approach to assess the mass relative to surrounding intra- and extra-cardiac structures, tissue characterization, perfusion to assess for vascularity

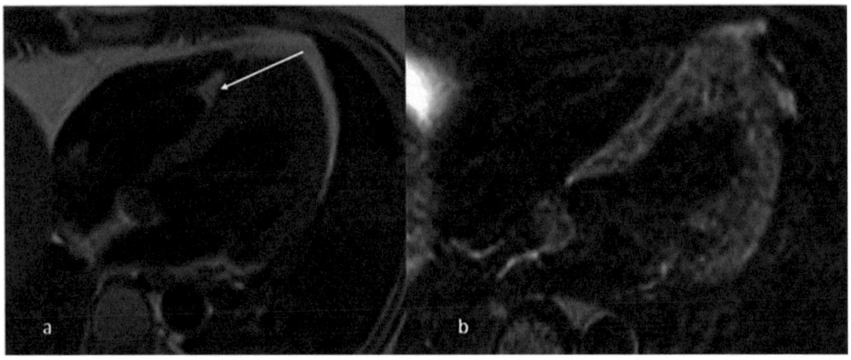

Figure 14.
T2 Stir image without (a) and with (b) fat saturation, showing a fatty mass in the right ventricular apex, likely lipoma.

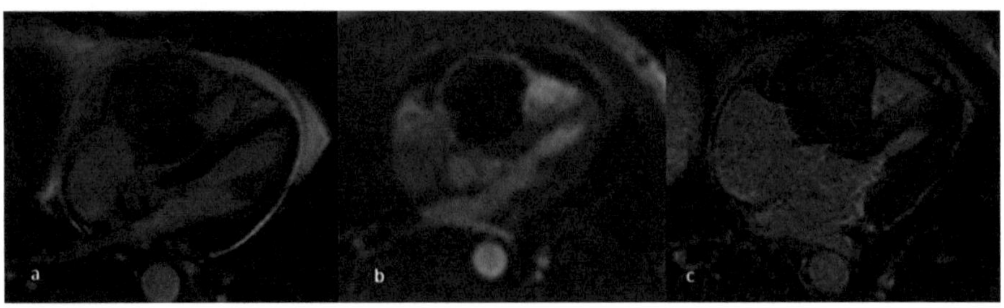

Figure 15.
Four-chamber cine (a), perfusion (b) and DE (c) imaging in a large RV mass showing a large mass, which has partial perfusion, and a partial "etched appearance" on DE imaging consistent with a tumor with a large thrombus burden.

and enhancement. CMR enables the evaluation of various characteristics including morphology, dimensions, location, extension, homogeneity, presence of infiltration in the surrounding tissues, and signal characteristics that aid in histopathological characterization. These signal characteristics encompass fatty infiltration, necrosis, hemorrhage, calcification, vascularity, among others. To achieve a comprehensive assessment, several imaging sequences are employed, such as double-inversion recovery fast spin-echo with triple inversion recovery to assess the amount of fat within the mass, (**Figure 14**) pre-contrast T2-weighted imaging, resting first-pass perfusion sequences, early gadolinium imaging, and late gadolinium DE imaging (**Figure 15**) [40]. CMR is considered a non-invasive biopsy in the assessment of cardiac masses.

4.5 Pericardial evaluation

CMR is a highly beneficial tool for evaluating and tracking various pericardial conditions, such as pericarditis, pericardial effusion, and constrictive pericarditis. Cine sequences evaluate function and effusion, free-breathing real time sequence assess ventricular interdependence in constriction, T2-STIR identifies edema, DE sequence detects LGE that indicates inflammation or fibrosis (**Figure 16**), and other T1- and T2-weighted and perfusion imaging techniques are used for tissue characterization of pericardial effusion and masses [41]. DE sequence plays a crucial role

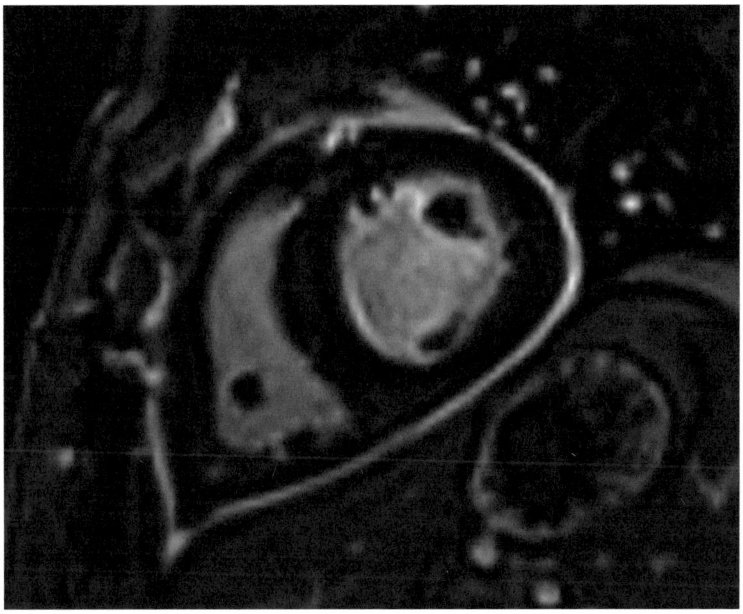

Figure 16.
Short axis DE imaging showing diffuse circumferential pericardial enhancement, consistent with acute pericarditis.

in diagnosing pericardial inflammation and monitoring the effectiveness of anti-inflammatory treatments [42]. The degree of pericardial LGE observed in the initial MRI is significantly linked to recurring episodes of pericarditis and the need for intensified therapy. Recent research has introduced quantitative methods for measuring pericardial LGE, which may have potential clinical applications in the future [43]. Differentiating between active pericarditis and chronic inflammation leading to constrictive pericarditis is of utmost importance, as the treatment modalities are completely different (anti-inflammatory drugs vs. pericardiectomy).

4.6 Arrhythmias and application in electrophysiology

CMR is widely used in electrophysiology (EP) for primary prevention of SCD and for secondary prevention in both brady and tachy arrhythmias. ICDs are used for primary prevention of SCD in patients with ischemic and NICM. A proportion of these patients do not have any lethal arrhythmias after implantation, prompting the need for better risk stratification of these patients. Scar quantification by DE imaging has been shown to have prognostic value in identifying patients more likely to benefit from ICD implantation for primary prevention. Further studies are underway to identify percent of scar and features of scar which denote increased arrhythmogenic substrate. CMR adds significantly to the management of patients presenting with bradyarrhythmia and heart block. Identification of scar involving the myocardium, predominantly the basal septum has been seen with cardiac sarcoidosis in addition to other etiologies.

Patients presenting with arrhythmias causing SCD from a variety of etiologies benefit from a CMR to identify and understand myocardial characteristics and abnormalities. In patients with arrhythmias, mapping techniques, such as T1/T2, can identify edema, necrosis, and scarring contributing to arrhythmias [44] which is further enhanced by identification of LGE in DE imaging. Further characterization of these lesions and anatomical geometry with CMR also allows for stratifying patients most suitable for ablation [45], along with identifying focus of arrhythmia to assist with ablation procedures. These maps can be used alone or integrated with electro-anatomic mapping to identify potential arrhythmogenic targets for ablation [46]. Post-ablation CMR images can also be used to determine prognostic factors contributing to the recurrence of arrhythmia.

Real-time CMR ablations have also been studied as an alternative to current ablation procedures utilizing radiation and iodinated contrast [47]; however, clinical implementation is limited by a lack of CMR-compatible devices and catheters required for these procedures.

4.7 Congenital heart disease (CHD)

In CHD, CMR can aid in diagnostics as well as post-intervention follow up. CMR provides unrestricted evaluation of intracardiac and vascular structures pertinent to the altered anatomy present in CHD to assist with diagnosis. Assessment of LV and RV size and function by cine, shunt quantification and Qp/Qs calculations by flow hemodynamics assist in assessing the severity of congenital heart defect guiding medical and surgical management accordingly (**Figure 17**). The utilization of contrast enhanced MRA is highly advantageous in visualizing and defining vascular structures, which often exhibit abnormalities in cases of CHD [48]. CMR is considered the imaging modality of choice in the serial follow in CHD.

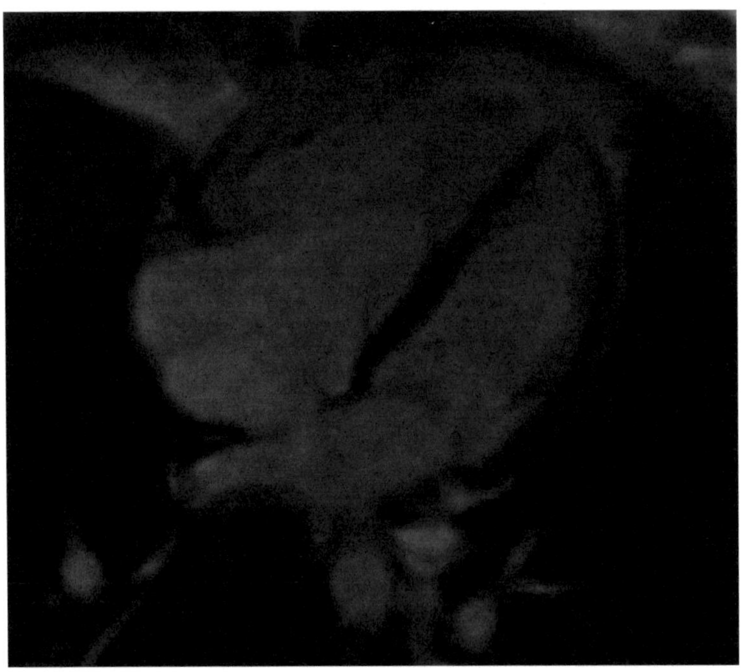

Figure 17.
Four chamber cine showing defect in the atrial septum with dilated right atrium and ventricle in a patient with atrial septal defect.

5. Advances in CMR

Advances are being made in CMR in the scanning part and in post processing. This section discusses technologic developments and advances in CMR with a focus on improvements in data acquisition, and reconstruction, new technologies and new clinical applications of CMR, MR guided cardiac procedures, and the role of artificial intelligence and machine learning in further advancing the field.

5.1 Advances in data acquisition techniques

5.1.1 Faster scanning

One of the limitations for the widespread use of CMR has been the time needed for scanning and for post processing. Considerable efforts are underway to decrease these times with a focus on improving the speed and efficiency of image acquisition, resolution, and reconstruction. Parallel imaging (PI) is used currently to decrease acquisition times. PI reduces redundant phase coiling data and processing steps [49]. PI, however, has known limitations due to under-sampling, such as lowering the signal-to-noise ratio and thus contributing to image degradation [50]. A novel method has since been developed called compressed sensing (CS) that utilizes similar under-sampling from PI with the addition of a noise-reduction algorithm [51]. CS results in faster data acquisition times without compromising image quality [51]. Current research is directed at further optimizing these systems to improve image quality and reduce artifacts, such as combing CS and PI [52] and designing algorithms to separate cardiac and respiration motion artifacts [53]. In addition to developments with CS, there is an interest in implementing artificial intelligence (AI) to improve data acquisition and processing performance further. The use of deep learning (DL) has been shown to accurately reconstruct cardiac MRI images at a faster rate compared to the methods described previously [54].

5.1.2 Respiratory and cardiac gating

Respiratory and cardiac gating techniques are well-established with CMR to reduce the physiologic motion of both systems and synchronize data acquisition throughout the cardiorespiratory cycle. These gating methods rely on ECGs, and image accuracy can be affected by arrhythmia and fluctuations in cardiac rhythm even in healthy subjects [55]. Novel techniques have been developed, such as non-ECG gated protocols, and have been found to improve spatial resolution and reduce cardiac motion artifacts without relying on ECG synchronization [56]. The same techniques have been implemented to reduce respiratory motion artifacts [57].

5.1.3 Whole heart spatial coverage

One of the limitations of current CMR imaging protocols is the use of 2D mapping slices. This method limits image acquisition to focal areas of tissue due to the thicker slices that can only cover a portion of the heart and require multiple breath holds impractical for certain patient populations. Newer mapping techniques have now emerged that provide a comprehensive analysis and image of the entire heart to better detect fibrosis and edema that may have been missed on older scanning modalities. This developing image acquisition technique provides whole heart spatial coverage with 3-dimensional (3D) data from one scan. The quicker scan times and improvements in motion artifacts have allowed for whole heart spatial coverage with 3D analysis to emerge as an effective alternative to more invasive diagnostic imaging techniques. While the image quality is currently a limitation, further efforts are in progress with potential in this area.

5.1.4 Cardiac mapping

Myocardial mapping and CMR fingerprinting continue to expand. Data acquisition speed and accuracy improvements have expanded the clinical utility of T1 and T2 mapping. CMR fingerprinting has recently been developed to efficiently produce T1 and T2 maps from a single scan and single breath hold [58]. Additional uses have included measuring fat fraction to further characterize ischemic scars to better prognosticate cardiomyopathies [59]. Future progression is focused on applying fingerprinting to more advanced imaging sequences in 3-dimensional (3D) and 4-dimensional (4D) data sets.

5.2 Stress testing

While stress testing is commonly used, the predominant form of stress is chemical. The difficulty with treadmill stress is the expense involved with MRI compatible treadmills along with the need to lay the patient down quickly on the MRI scanning table in the same position as images obtained prior to stress. Another limitation is excess motion whether whole body or during respiration with exercise. A novel stress testing technique is supine MRI-compatible exercise ergometer. With a better safety profile than pharmacological stressors, physical stress on the heart visualized via CMR can provide insight into tissue function and characteristics specific to ischemia [60]. For post processing of stress perfusion sequences, currently most centers use visual estimation for stress perfusion. Current quantitative perfusion post processing software is tedious and time consuming. Advances are being made in stress testing with faster post processing software for quantitative perfusion.

5.3 Artifact reduction

Artifact reduction has become important to obtain CMR images in patients with pacemakers (PM) and ICDs. Despite developments in manufacturing MRI-compatible PM and ICDs, there remains difficulty in acquiring accurate CMR images of the myocardium due to the obscuring metal artifacts from these devices [61]. Inversion recovery sequences in LGE imaging have since been modified by adjusting the bandwidth and rate of pulsed radio frequencies to eliminate hyperintense artifacts [62]. These efforts have further expanded compatible patient populations who may benefit from CMR.

5.4 4-dimensional (4D) acquisition

Four-dimensional (4D) data acquisition especially for flow analysis is an emerging advanced imaging sequence in CMR. The data from 4D image reconstruction provides 3D dynamic values over time, which can be useful in patients with complex anatomy and differing flow gradients [57]. While clinical application of 4D image acquisition is limited by a lack of ubiquitous hardware and software, there is vast potential in developing imaging protocols to better diagnose and monitor valvular pathologies and CHD.

5.5 Myocardial strain

While myocardial strain is being done by TTE currently, the use of CMR strain has significant potential (**Figure 18**). Myocardial strain assesses myocardial deformation and can serve as a precursor to myocardial dysfunction and cardiomyopathy [64] and has also been shown to predict cardiac mortality [65]. CMR is emerging as a diagnostic modality in determining myocardial strain due to several developing techniques. Displacement encoding with stimulated echocardiography (DENSE) is an acquisition method that measures myocardial tissue displacement to estimate strain. Feature tracking (FT) is another post-processing algorithm that calculates myocardial deformation [66]. Both DENSE and FT have been utilized to measure cardiac strain. However, a lack of inter-vendor standardization and clinical validity for cardiac strain remain salient limitations [66]. A new and developing technique called fast strain-encoded CMR (fast-SENC) is another imaging technique that can determine cardiac contractility with comparable results to FT and DENSE [67]. The clinical implication

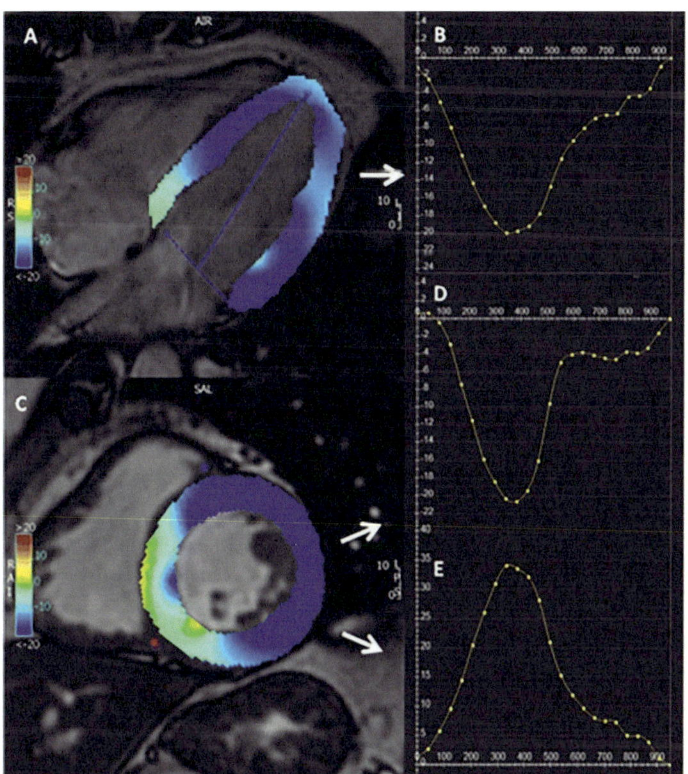

Figure 18.
Example of colored strain analysis with a feature-tracking software (Circle CVI42®). From long-axis four-chamber SSFP cine image (a), longitudinal strain curve is derived (b) and short-axis SSFP image (c) is used for calculation of circumferential (d) and radial strain curves (e). Reproduced with permission from Scatteia et al. [63].

is evaluating subclinical cardiomyopathies and adjusting treatment plans to prevent or monitor disease progression.

5.6 Diffusion-weighted CMR

Clinical utility and advances in diffusion-weighted imaging (DWI) of the heart is evolving. A subcategory of cardiac DWI with clinical potential is diffusion tensor imaging (DTI). DTI allows for 3-dimensional visualization and diffusion parameters of the cardiomyocyte microstructure without the need for exogenous contrast [68]. This modality measures water diffusion gradients within myocytes that are reconstructed to provide information about myofibers' orientation, rotation, and torsion [32]. One limitation of DWI and DTI in the heart is the signal loss inherent with cardiac motion which prevents the identification of true signal loss due to diffusion compared to signal loss due to cardiac motion. Recent advances have augmented pre-existing algorithms to account for this motion discrepancy [69] and improvements in the DTI data acquisition process reduce the total imaging time [70]. While the clinical utility of DTI information continues to expand, multiple studies have investigated how the cardiac microstructure data is affected by various pathologies. Parameters such as myocyte fiber orientation, fractional anisotropy, mean diffusivity gradients, tractographic propagation angle, and helical angle are all novel approaches to better characterizing infarcted tissue [71].

5.7 CMR guided interventions

CMR-guided interventions are continuously developing. Procedures like percutaneous coronary intervention used for obstructive CAD can cause acute kidney injury from the iodinated contrast used, leading to an increase in all-cause mortality [72]. Additionally, fluoroscopy exposes patients and staff to ionized radiation, increasing the risk of future malignancy [73]. While fluoroscopic X-ray remains the gold standard for these procedures, there is growing interest in using cardiac MRI as a procedural aid to reduce the need for fluoroscopy. Transarterial valve replacements and stenting procedures using CMR have been utilized in animal studies, however, the feasibility of implementing these techniques in human subjects remains a challenge and is still experimental at this stage. Other interventional cardiac procedures have also utilized CMR to reduce their fluoroscopic footprint such as EP.

5.8 Artificial intelligence and machine learning

Artificial intelligence (AI) is quickly becoming one of the fastest-growing fields within CMR. Briefly, AI is the method of developing intelligent algorithms that can perform tasks and solve complex problems [74]. Machine learning (ML) is a subset of AI that continually improves pattern recognition and makes data inferences with the more data it processes [75]. Although the clinical applications of AI and ML are still being developed and validated, implementing these resources will drastically change the future of CMR. Most notably, AI will significantly contribute to data acquisition and reconstruction acceleration, expand CMR metrics for further diagnostic and therapeutic effects, and increase the accessibility of CMR [75]. The current ML systems that have been developed expand on CS data acquisition models to further reconstruct under-sampled data. These models learn from CMR data sets by further exploiting redundancies of the temporospatial relationships of tissue, thus resulting in quicker processing times and equivocal imaging resolution [75]. There have been numerous examples of ML-generated systems significantly accelerating processing times in CMR angiography [75], whole heart 3D LGE reconstruction [76], reduction of respiratory motion artifact [77], and T1 and T2 mapping [78]. Intracardiac volume measurements have also been generated from ML systems and have been used to risk stratify patients with severe AS [79]. There are instances where ML has been found to be more accurate in measuring certain parameters, such as ventricular volume, compared to human analyses [80]. Newer approaches are using ML to identify ischemic scars without utilizing LGE CMR and subjecting patients to contrast [81]. The clinical use of ML continues to expand within all fields of CMR in identifying fibrosis and scar with and without LGE, 3D and 4D flow reconstruction, and mapping techniques.

Several limitations exist regarding ML in CMR, given the field's novelty. For one, ML requires a fully sampled learning database to make inferences on testing samples, which is not widely available. Evidence suggests variations in image reconstruction based on certain parameters from the learning database, such as signal-to-noise ratios [82]. Additional improvements in central and graphical processing units are required to run these systems and models. Despite these restrictions, the use of AI and ML in CMR continues to improve and may have significant implications in imaging accessibility by providing automated analyses of cardiac disease.

6. Conclusion

CMR is an excellent and comprehensive imaging modality, providing information about myocardial structure, function, tissue characterization, edema, infiltration, inflammation, scar, myocardial perfusion, congenital heart disease, shunts, flow quantification in addition to viability and any other cardiac abnormalities like masses. Currently being limited by the time involved in acquiring the scan and in the post processing of these scans, as seen above, there are a lot of advances and research happening in all areas. The clinical and research uses of CMR continue to grow and it continues to offer valuable insight into a variety of cardiac pathologies.

Acknowledgements

All three authors had substantial contribution to the book chapter writing in drafting, revising the work and approval of the manuscript version to be published. The authors would like to acknowledge Michaela Kiel, Medical student for her assistance in the initial stages of the work.

Author details

Hunter Frederiksen, Corina Iorgoveanu and Mahi L. Ashwath*
University of Iowa Hospitals and Clinics, University of Iowa, Iowa City, USA

*Address all correspondence to: mahi-ashwath@uiowa.edu

References

[1] Leiner T, Bogaert J, Friedrich MG, Mohiaddin R, Muthurangu V, Myerson S, et al. On clinical indications for cardiovascular magnetic resonance. Journal of Cardiovascular Magnetic Resonance. 2020;**22**:1-37

[2] Kuruvilla S, Adenaw N, Katwal AB, Lipinski MJ, Kramer CM, Salerno M. Late gadolinium enhancement on cardiac magnetic resonance predicts adverse cardiovascular outcomes in nonischemic cardiomyopathy: A systematic review and meta-analysis. Circulation. Cardiovascular Imaging. 2014;**7**:250-257

[3] Haaf P, Garg P, Messroghli DR, Broadbent DA, Greenwood JP, Plein S. Cardiac T1 mapping and extracellular volume (ECV) in clinical practice: A comprehensive review. Journal of Cardiovascular Magnetic Resonance. 2016;**18**:1-12

[4] Centers for Disease Control and Prevention. CDC WONDER: Multiple Cause of Death. https://wonder.cdc.gov/mcd.html. 2023

[5] Nagel E, Greenwood JP, McCann GP, Bettencourt N, Shah AM, Hussain ST, et al. Magnetic resonance perfusion or fractional flow Reserve in Coronary Disease. New England Journal. 2019;**380**:2418-2428

[6] Wu KC, Zerhouni EA, Judd RM, Lugo-Olivieri H, Barouch LA, et al. Prognostic significance of microvascular obstruction by magnetic resonance imaging in patients with acute myocardial infarction. Circulation. 1998;**97**:765-772

[7] Kim RJ, Wu E, Rafael A, Chen E-L, Parker MA, Simonetti O, et al. The use of contrast-enhanced magnetic resonance imaging to identify reversible myocardial dysfunction. New England Journal. 2000;**343**:1445-1453

[8] Srichai MB, Junor C, Rodriguez LL, Stillman AE, Grimm RA, Lieber ML, et al. Clinical, imaging, and pathological characteristics of left ventricular thrombus: A comparison of contrast-enhanced magnetic resonance imaging, transthoracic echocardiography, and transesophageal echocardiography with surgical or pathological validation. American Heart Journal. 2006;**152**:75-84

[9] Goyal P, Weinsaft JW. Cardiovascular magnetic resonance imaging for cardiac Thrombus. Methodist DeBakey Cardiovascular Journal. 2013;**9**:132-136

[10] Wagner A, Mahrholdt H, Holly TA, Elliott MD, Regenfus M, Parker M, et al. Contrast-enhanced MRI and routine single photon emission computed tomography (SPECT) perfusion imaging for detection of subendocardial myocardial infarcts: An imaging study. The Lancet. 2003;**361**:374-379

[11] Al-Sabeq B, Nabi F, Shah DJ. Assessment of myocardial viability by cardiac MRI. Current Opinion in Cardiology. 2019;**34**:502-509

[12] Kim HW, Klem I, Shah DJ, Wu E, Meyers SN, Parker MA, et al. Unrecognized non-Q-wave myocardial infarction: Prevalence and prognostic significance in patients with suspected coronary disease. PLoS Medicine. 2009;**6**

[13] Kolentinis M, Le M, Nagel E, Puntmann VO. Contemporary cardiac MRI in chronic coronary artery

disease. European Cardiology Review. 2020;**2020**:15

[14] Greenwood JP, Mbchb M, Younger JF, Ball SG, Radjenovic A, Ma B, et al. Cardiovascular magnetic resonance and single-photon emission computed tomography for diagnosis of coronary heart disease (CE-MARC): A prospective trial. The Lancet. 2012;**379**:453-460

[15] Kwong RY, Ge Y, Steel K, Bingham S, Abdullah S, Fujikura K, et al. Cardiac magnetic resonance stress perfusion imaging for evaluation of patients with chest pain. Journal of the American College of Cardiology. 2019;**74**:1741-1755

[16] Patel AR, Salerno M, Kwong RY, Singh A, Heydari B, Kramer CM. Stress cardiac magnetic resonance myocardial perfusion imaging: JACC review topic of the week. Journal of the American College of Cardiology. 2021;**78**:1655-1668

[17] Feger J, Sam D. Hypertrophic Cardiomyopathy. https://radiopaedia.org/articles/hypertrophic-cardiomyopathy?lang=us. 2009

[18] Chan RH, Maron BJ, Olivotto I, Pencina MJ, Assenza GE, Haas T, et al. Prognostic value of quantitative contrast-enhanced cardiovascular magnetic resonance for the evaluation of sudden death risk in patients with hypertrophic cardiomyopathy. Circulation. 2014;**130**:484-495

[19] Malik N, Mukherjee M, Wu KC, Zimmerman SL, Zhan J, Calkins H, et al. Multimodality imaging in Arrhythmogenic right ventricular cardiomyopathy. Circulation. Cardiovascular Imaging. 2022;**15**:e013725

[20] Petersen SE, Jensen B, Aung N, Friedrich MG, McMahon CJ, Mohiddin SA, et al. Excessive Trabeculation of the left ventricle: JACC: Cardiovascular imaging expert panel paper. JACC: Cardiovascular Imaging. 2023;**16**:408-425

[21] Zuccarino F, Vollmer I, Sanchez G, Navallas M, Pugliese F, Gayete A. Left ventricular noncompaction: Imaging findings and diagnostic criteria. American Journal of Roentgenology. 2015;**204**:W519-W530

[22] Bruder O, Wagner A, Lombardi M, Schwitter J, Van Rossum A, Pilz G, et al. European cardiovascular magnetic resonance (EuroCMR) registry – Multi national results from 57 centers in 15 countries. Journal of Cardiovascular Magnetic Resonance. 2013;**15**:1-9

[23] Abdel-Aty H, Boyé P, Zagrosek A, Wassmuth R, Kumar A, Messroghli D, et al. Diagnostic performance of cardiovascular magnetic resonance in patients with suspected acute myocarditis: Comparison of different approaches. Journal of the American College of Cardiology. 2005;**45**: 1815-1822

[24] Ferreira VM, Piechnik SK, Dall'Armellina E, Karamitsos TD, Francis JM, Ntusi N, et al. Native T1-mapping detects the location, extent and patterns of acute myocarditis without the need for gadolinium contrast agents. Journal of Cardiovascular Magnetic Resonance. 2014;**16**:1-11

[25] Anand S, Janardhanan R. Role of cardiac MRI in nonischemic cardiomyopathies. Indian Heart Journal. 2016;**68**:405-409

[26] Syed IS, Glockner JF, Feng DL, Araoz PA, Martinez MW, Edwards WD, et al. Role of cardiac magnetic resonance imaging in the detection of cardiac amyloidosis. JACC: Cardiovascular Imaging. 2010;**3**:155-164

[27] Austin BA, Tang WHW, Rodriguez ER, Tan C, Flamm SD,

Taylor DO, et al. Delayed hyper-enhancement magnetic resonance imaging provides incremental diagnostic and prognostic utility in suspected cardiac amyloidosis. JACC: Cardiovascular Imaging. 2009;**2**:1369-1377

[28] Schelbert EB, Messroghli DR. State of the art: Clinical applications of cardiac T1 mapping. Radiology. 2016;**278**:658-676

[29] Tavora F, Cresswell N, Li L, Ripple M, Solomon C, Burke A. Comparison of necropsy findings in patients with sarcoidosis dying suddenly from cardiac sarcoidosis versus dying suddenly from other causes. The American Journal of Cardiology. 2009;**104**:571-577

[30] Patel M, Cawley PJ, Heitner JF, Klem I, Parker MA, Jaroudi WA, et al. Detection of myocardial damage in patients with sarcoidosis. Circulation. 2009;**120**:1969-1977

[31] Lee E, Ibrahim E-SH, Parwani P, Bhave N, Stojanovska J. Practical guide to evaluating myocardial disease by cardiac MRI. American Journal of Roentgenology. 2020;**214**:546-556

[32] Patel AR, Rashedi N. Cardiac sarcoidosis: A picture may be worth a thousand words, but do we need more? Journal of the American Heart Association. 2019;**8**:1-3

[33] Azevedo O, Cordeiro F, Gago MF, Miltenberger-miltenyi G, Ferreira C, Sousa N, et al. Fabry disease and the heart: A comprehensive review. International Journal of Molecular Sciences. 2021;**22**:1-36

[34] Tower-Rader A, Jaber WA. Multimodality imaging assessment of Fabry disease. Circulation. Cardiovascular Imaging. 2019;**12**:1-13

[35] Abdel-Gadir A, Treibel T, Moon J. Myocardial T1 mapping: Where are we now and where are we going? Research reports. Clinical Cardiology. 2014;**339**:339-347

[36] Espinoza Romero C, Lima ICV, Hotta VT, Bocchi EA, Salemi VMC. Endomyocardial fibrosis of the right ventricle in a patient with schistosomiasis: A case report. European Heart Journal Case Report. 2022;**6**:1-6

[37] Carvalho FP, Azevedo CF. Comprehensive assessment of endomyocardial fibrosis with cardiac MRI: Morphology, function, and tissue characterization. Radiographics. 2020;**40**:336-353

[38] Cawley PJ, Maki JH, Otto CM. Cardiovascular magnetic resonance imaging for valvular heart disease technique and validation. Circulation. 2009;**119**:468-478

[39] Gatti M, D'Angelo T, Muscogiuri G, Dell'aversana S, Andreis A, Carisio A, et al. Cardiovascular magnetic resonance of cardiac tumors and masses. World Journal of Cardiology. 2021;**13**:628-649

[40] Tyebally S, Chen D, Bhattacharyya S, Mughrabi A, Hussain Z, Manisty C, et al. Cardiac Tumors: JACC CardioOncology state-of-the-art review. JACC CardioOncol. 2020;**2**:293-311

[41] Wang TKM. Clinical applications of cardiac magnetic resonance imaging in pericardial diseases. American College of Cardiology, Latest in Cardiology. 2023. Accessed from: https://www.acc.org/Latest-in-Cardiology/Articles/2022/08/10/12/06/Clinical-Applications-of-Cardiac-MRI-in-Pericardial-Diseases

[42] Chetrit M, Xu B, Kwon DH, Ramchand J, Rodriguez RE, Tan CD, et al. Imaging-guided therapies for pericardial diseases. JACC: Cardiovascular Imaging. 2020;**13**:1422-1437

[43] Kumar A, Sato K, Yzeiraj E, Betancor J, Lin L, Tamarappoo BK, et al. Quantitative pericardial delayed hyperenhancement informs clinical course in recurrent pericarditis. JACC Cardiovasc Imaging. 2017;**10**:1337-1346

[44] Mont L, Roca-Luque I, Althoff TF. Ablation lesion assessment with MRI. Arrhythmic Electrophysiological Review. 2022;**11**:1-11

[45] Marrouche NF, Wilber D, Hindricks G, Jais P, Akoum N, Marchlinski F, et al. Association of atrial tissue fibrosis identified by delayed enhancement MRI and atrial fibrillation catheter ablation: The DECAAF study. JAMA. 2014;**311**:498-506

[46] Bisbal F, Guiu E, Cabanas-Grandío P, Berruezo A, Prat-Gonzalez S, Vidal B, et al. CMR-guided approach to localize and ablate gaps in repeat AF ablation procedure. JACC Cardiovasc Imaging. 2014;**7**:653-663

[47] Toupin S, Bour P, Lepetit-Coiffé M, Ozenne V, Denis de Senneville B, Schneider R, et al. Feasibility of real-time MR thermal dose mapping for predicting radiofrequency ablation outcome in the myocardium in vivo. Journal of Cardiovascular Magnetic Resonance. 2017;**19**:1-12

[48] Pushparajah K, Duong P, Mathur S, Babu-Narayan SV. Cardiovascular MRI and CT in congenital heart disease. Echo Research Practice. 2019;**6**:R121-R138

[49] Jaspan ON, Fleysher R, Lipton ML. Compressed sensing MRI: A review of the clinical literature. British Journal of Radiology. 2015;**88**:1-12

[50] Glockner JF, Hu HH, Stanley DW, Angelos L, King K. Parallel MR imaging: A user's guide. Radiographics. 2005;**25**:1279-1297

[51] Curione D, Ciliberti P, Monti CB, Capra D, Bordonaro V, Ciancarella P, et al. Compressed sensing cardiac cine imaging compared with standard balanced steady-state free precession cine imaging in a Pediatric population. Radiological Cardiothoracic Imaging. 2022;**4**:1-9

[52] Hu Z, Zhao C, Zhao X, Kong L, Yang J, Wang X, et al. Joint reconstruction framework of compressed sensing and nonlinear parallel imaging for dynamic cardiac magnetic resonance imaging. BMC Medical Imaging. 2021;**21**:1-14

[53] Feng L, Axel L, Chandarana H, Block KT, Sodickson DK, Otazo R. XD-GRASP: Golden-angle radial MRI with reconstruction of extra motion-state dimensions using compressed sensing. Magnetic Resonance in Medicine. 2016;**75**:775-788

[54] Bustin A, Fuin N, Botnar RM, Prieto C. From compressed-sensing to artificial intelligence-based cardiac MRI reconstruction. Frontier in Cardiovascular Medicine. 2020;**7**:1-19

[55] Menchón-Lara RM, Simmross-Wattenberg F, Casaseca-de-la-Higuera P, Martín-Fernández M, Alberola-López C. Reconstruction techniques for cardiac cine MRI. Insights Imaging. 2019;**10**:1-16

[56] Sharif B, Arsanjani R, Dharmakumar R, Bairey Merz CN, Berman DS, Li D. All-systolic non-ECG-gated myocardial perfusion MRI:

Feasibility of multi-slice continuous first-pass imaging. Magnetic Resonance in Medicine. 2015;**74**:1661-1674

[57] Pennig L, Lennartz S, Wagner A, Sokolowski M, Gajzler M, Ney S, et al. Clinical application of free-breathing 3D whole heart late gadolinium enhancement cardiovascular magnetic resonance with high isotropic spatial resolution using compressed SENSE. Journal of Cardiovascular Magnetic Resonance. 2020;**22**:1-13

[58] Cavallo AU, Liu Y, Patterson A, Al-Kindi S, Hamilton J, Gilkeson R, et al. CMR fingerprinting for myocardial T1, T2, and ECV quantification in patients with nonischemic cardiomyopathy. JACC: Cardiovascular Imaging. 2019;**12**:1584-1585

[59] Jaubert O, Cruz G, Bustin A, Hajhosseiny R, Nazir S, Schneider T, et al. T1, T2, and fat fraction cardiac MR fingerprinting: Preliminary clinical evaluation. Journal of Magnetic Resonance Imaging. 2021;**53**:1253-1265

[60] He B, Chen Y, Wang L, Yang Y, Xia C, Zheng J, et al. Compact MR-compatible ergometer and its application in cardiac MR under exercise stress: A preliminary study. Magnetic Resonance in Medicine. 2022;**88**:1927-1936

[61] Sasaki T, Hansford R, Zviman MM, Kolandaivelu A, Bluemke DA, Berger RD, et al. Quantitative Assessment of Artifacts on Cardiac Magnetic Resonance Imaging of Patients with Pacemakers and Implantable Cardioverter-Defibrillators. Circ Cardiovasc Imaging. 2011;**4**:662-670

[62] Ibrahim E-SH, Runge M, Stojanovska J, Agarwal P, Ghadimi-Mahani M, Attili A, et al. Optimized cardiac magnetic resonance imaging inversion recovery sequence for metal artifact reduction and accurate myocardial scar assessment in patients with cardiac implantable electronic devices. World Journal de Radiologie. 2018;**10**:100-107

[63] Scatteia A, Baritussio A, Bucciarelli-Ducci C. Strain imaging using cardiac magnetic resonance. Heart Failure Review. 2017;**22**:465-476

[64] Montenbruck M, Kelle S, Esch S, Schwarz AK, Giusca S, Korosoglou G, et al. Hypertension-hypertension-diagnostic methods CMR fast-SENC segmental intramyocardial LV strain monitors decline in heart function before ejection fraction in patient with arterial hypertension. European Heart Journal. 2020;**41**:2748

[65] Luis SA, Chan J, Pellikka PA. Echocardiographic assessment of left ventricular systolic function: An overview of contemporary techniques, including speckle-tracking echocardiography. Mayo Clinic Proceeding. 2019;**94**:125-138

[66] Backhaus SJ, Metschies G, Billing M, Kowallick JT, Gertz RJ, Lapinskas T, et al. Cardiovascular magnetic resonance imaging feature tracking: Impact of training on observer performance and reproducibility. PLoS One. 2019;**14**:1-16

[67] Siry D, Riffel J, Salatzki J, André F, Weberling LD, Ochs M, et al. A head-to-head comparison of fast-SENC and feature tracking to LV long axis strain for assessment of myocardial deformation in chest pain patients. BMC Medical Imaging. 2022;**22**:1-17

[68] Khalique Z, Ferreira PF, Scott AD, Nielles-Vallespin S, Firmin DN, Pennell DJ. Diffusion tensor cardiovascular magnetic resonance imaging: A clinical perspective. JACC: Cardiovascular Imaging. 2020;**13**:1235-1255

[69] Delattre BMA, Viallon M, Wei H, Zhu YM, Feiweier T, Pai VM, et al. In vivo cardiac diffusion-weighted magnetic resonance imaging: Quantification of normal perfusion and diffusion coefficients with intravoxel incoherent motion imaging. Investigative Radiology. 2012;**47**:662-670

[70] McClymont D, Teh I, Whittington HJ, Grau V, Schneider JE. Prospective acceleration of diffusion tensor imaging with compressed sensing using adaptive dictionaries. Magnetic Resonance in Medicine. 2016;**76**:248-258

[71] Wu MT, Su MY, Huang YL, Chiou KR, Yang P, Pan H, et al. Sequential changes of myocardial microstructure in patients postmyocardial infarction by diffusion-tensor cardiac MR correlation with left ventricular structure and function. Circulation. Cardiovascular Imaging. 2009;**2**:32-40

[72] Tsai TT, Patel UD, Chang TI, Kennedy KF, Masoudi FA, Matheny ME, et al. Contemporary incidence, predictors, and outcomes of acute kidney injury in patients undergoing percutaneous coronary interventions: Insights from the NCDR cath-PCI registry. JACC. Cardiovascular Interventions. 2014;7:1-9

[73] Partridge J. Radiation in the cardiac catheter laboratory. Heart. 2005;**91**:1615-1620

[74] Leiner T, Rueckert D, Suinesiaputra A, Baeßler B, Nezafat R, Išgum I, et al. Machine learning in cardiovascular magnetic resonance: Basic concepts and applications. Journal of Cardiovascular Magnetic Resonance. 2019;**21**:1-14

[75] Fotaki A, Puyol-Antón E, Chiribiri A, Botnar R, Pushparajah K, Prieto C. Artificial intelligence in cardiac MRI: Is clinical adoption forthcoming? Frontier in Cardiovascular Medicine. 2022;**8**:1-13

[76] Kamesh Iyer S, Tasdizen T, Burgon N, Kholmovski E, Marrouche N, Adluru G, et al. Compressed sensing for rapid late gadolinium enhanced imaging of the left atrium: A preliminary study. Magnetic Resonance Imaging. 2016;**34**:846-854

[77] Weiger M, Börnert P, Proksa R, Schäffter T, Haase A. Motion-adapted gating based on k-space weighting for reduction of respiratory motion artifacts. Magnetic Resonance in Medicine. 1997;**38**:322-333

[78] Hamilton JI, Currey D, Rajagopalan S, Seiberlich N. Deep learning reconstruction for cardiac magnetic resonance fingerprinting T1 and T2 mapping. Magnetic Resonance in Medicine. 2021;**85**:2127-2135

[79] Evertz R, Lange T, Backhaus SJ, Schulz A, Beuthner BE, Topci R, et al. Artificial intelligence enabled fully automated CMR function quantification for optimized risk stratification in patients undergoing Transcatheter aortic valve replacement. Journal of Interventional Cardiology. 2022;**2022**:1-9

[80] Alabed S, Alandejani F, Dwivedi K, Karunasaagarar K, Sharkey M, Garg P, et al. Validation of artificial intelligence cardiac MRI measurements: Relationship to heart catheterization and mortality prediction. Radiology. 2022;**305**:68-79

[81] Zhang Q, Burrage MK, Shanmuganathan M, Gonzales RA, Lukaschuk E, Thomas KE, et al. Artificial intelligence for contrast-free MRI: Scar assessment in myocardial infarction using deep learning-based virtual native enhancement. Circulation. 2022;**146**:1492-1503

[82] Knoll F, Hammernik K, Zhang C, Moeller S, Pock T, Sodickson DK, et al. Deep-learning methods for parallel magnetic resonance imaging reconstruction: A survey of the current approaches, trends, and issues. IEEE Signal Processing Magazine. 2020;**37**:128-140

Chapter 3

New Advances in Cardiac Magnetic Resonance Imaging of Congenital Heart Disease

Karima Hami

Abstract

Cardiac magnetic resonance (CMR) is an indispensable second-line tool, next to CT (computed tomography), in the evaluation and follow-up of congenital heart disease in adults and children, as a complement to echocardiography, without the inconvenience of X-rays. This imaging requires a long examination time and good cooperation from the patient to achieve good apnea, or the use of general anesthesia in children under 8 years of age. In this chapter, we summarize the recent advances in CMR sequences, notably the four-dimensional (4D) flow, in software and hardware technologies that allow a wider use, thanks to the simplification of the examination protocols and the decrease of the acquisition time.

Keywords: 4D flow, cardiovascular magnetic resonance, cardiac heart diseases, 3D printing, invasive CMR

1. Introduction

Significant improvements in the diagnosis and management of patients with congenital heart disease (CHD) have led to increased number of patients surviving to adulthood [1]. These patients require lifelong noninvasive follow-up to detect long-term complications [2, 3].

Since 2020, the ACC/AH and the ESC published [4] the new guidelines for the management of adult CHD [5].

CMR is the only imaging modality offering in a single time an excellent anatomical and functional information of the heart [6, 7]. Long follow-up with repetitive CMR imaging is reasonable for its high reproducibility and safety compared to CT and catheterization, in the young population.

This imaging requires a long examination time and good cooperation from the patient to achieve good apnea, or the use of general anesthesia in young children. The use of advanced CMR sequences as such a 4D flow is a good option for improving this limitation.

Novel emerging techniques especially advanced flow evaluation and reduced acquisition and post-processing times [8] are a major step forward in the evaluation of CHD with flow perturbations [9].

2. 4D flow

4D flow CMR refers to phase-contrast CMR with flow-encoding in all three spatial directions, in typical transverse, sagittal, and coronal planes and resolved to the three dimensions of space and the dimension of time along the cardiac cycle. It allows a velocity assessment in the whole heart and great vessels [10] with prospective or retrospective electrocardiogram (ECG) gating. The images obtained are displayed in a colored representation of the flow patterns.

The 4D flow enables a flow analysis in any vessel section in a single acquisition, which is especially relevant in complex CHD.

4D flow CMR requires a reliable ECG with detectable R-wave. To cover the entire aorta, it is important that the coils are positioned high enough to explore certain aortic pathologies. The scans can be relatively long and it is important to inform the patient before.

4D flow CMR employs spoiled gradient echo sequences with short TR for rapid imaging with the generation of PC angiograms without the need for an external contrast agent. According to the 4D flow cardiovascular magnetic resonance consensus statement 2023, the recommended spatial resolution in adult vessels is 2.5–3 mm^3, 2–2.5 mm^3 in pediatric vessels, and 30–50 ms for temporal resolution. A flip angle of 7° is advised if non-contrast acquisition [11].

The advantage of 4D flow CMR is the retrospective analysis of the blood flow through any planes of interest across the 3D volume.

Moreover, the analysis of advanced hemodynamic parameters as kinetic energy (KE) and wall shear stress (WSS) has become possible [12, 13].

4d flow allows precise assessment in a variety of clinical situations, including evaluation of the QP/QS ratio, collateral flow, and valve regurgitation.

Retrospective cardiac gating is preferred, to analyze the flow in systole and diastole.

Respiratory gating is used to avoid motion artifacts; respiratory motion compensation is a good alternative if it is available.

As with 2D, 4D flow requires a close value of real peak velocity to avoid aliasing. A VENC of 120–150 cm/s is sufficient in the absence of stenosis; otherwise it should be increased to the peak velocity expected by other methods, such as echocardiography, and using post-processing tools with anti-aliasing correction should be considered.

- Resolution: Acquired voxel size according to JCMR consensus document [11] for intracardiac flow is 3 mm or less. In small children, higher spatial resolution is recommended, because of the smaller FOV (field of view).

3. Application

3.1 Fontan repair

The Fontan operation is the last stage in the palliative treatment in univentricular heart [14].

The main goal of CMR is the assessment of the ventricle function, possible valvular regurgitation, the patency of the Fontan pathway, and the presence of collateral flow [15].

Various manifestations can occur such as protein-losing enteropathy, plastic bronchitis, interstitial pulmonary edema, pleuro-pericardial effusion, and ascites.

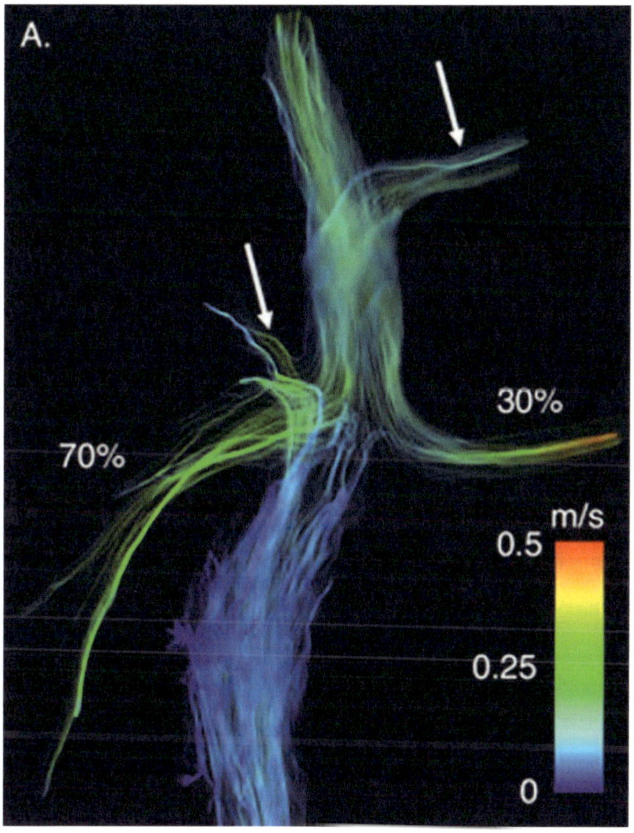

Figure 1.
4D flow MRI in a total cavo-pulmonary connection with flow distribution 70% into the RPA and 30% in LPA. RPA: Right pulmonary artery, LPA: Left pulmonary artery.

MR is able to characterize lymphatic perfusion abnormalities using static and dynamic sequences, which will not be detailed in this chapter.

Aortic forward flow should be equal to total systemic venous return and to total pulmonary venous return. The divergence in flows indicates the presence of regurgitant lesions, patent fenestration, or significant systemic-to-collateral [16].

Late gadolinium enhancement (LGE) imaging is indicated in cases of recent degradation in cardiac function, suspicion of thrombus formation, or new onset of complex arrhythmias to detect the presence and extension of myocardial fibrosis. Contrast-enhanced (CE-MRA) in the venous phase allows the assessment of the permeability of the Fontan circuit. Moreover, 4D flow imaging allows the quantification of any obstruction based on distribution patterns of caval or pulmonary artery flows (**Figure 1**) [16].

4. Tetralogy of Fallot (TOF)

An accurate assessment of pulmonary valve regurgitation (PVR) is essential prior to pulmonary revalvulation (PR). This assessment is better performed using 4D flow CMR because of the possibility to correct for through-plane motion of the valve and flow angulation. Advanced flow parameters such as ventricular kinetic energy

(KE) represent a novel tool to assess cardiac function; KE represents the amount of energy present in the blood flow due to movement and is considered a good marker of ventricular efficiency; it is calculated using the following equation: $KE = \frac{1}{2}mv^2$ where m represents the mass (the voxel volume multiplied by the density of blood) and v represents the velocity of each voxel, determined from the 4D flow. Jeong found that the KE was abnormal in TOF patients compared to in healthy controls [17].

According to the current CMR criteria, a large percentage of patients continue to experience symptoms of the classic complications observed in patients not undergoing PR, such us ventricular arrhythmias and heart failure [18].

4D flow provides a more accurate assessment of PV regurgitant flow, which may lead to better timing of revalvulation.

Several studies show that turbulent kinetic energy in the right ventricle was higher in patients with TOF than in healthy controls, mainly in the RVOT [17, 19, 20].

Jeong demonstrated that KE is an earlier indicator of cardiac dysfunction than classic parameters such us EDVI, ESVI, and EF.

Furthermore, patients with TOF may have pulmonary valve or branch stenosis. Consequently, analysis of PA flow based on 2D PC CMR plane is prone to error. Geiger and Francois [21] found that TOF patients present helical flow patterns in the pulmonary arteries [22].

These findings have been reported by Hu et al. [23]. They found that vortices were predominantly present in the main PA and helical flow patterns were predominantly present in the right PA, which was associated with systolic energy loss in the right PA and increased RV dimensions, suggesting impaired ventricular–arterial coupling.

5. Aortic diseases

In the aorta, aortic flow was assessed in all three segments, on the ascending, transverse, and descending aorta, in a plane perpendicular to the aortic axis.

The advantage of the 4D flow is that the plans can be placed after the acquisition.

Vorticity and helicity are two parameters that provide information about the rotational movement of blood flow.

Vorticity describes the rotation of a fluid particle around the same axis as well as around its own axis, which describes a curved movement.

Helicity is determined from vorticity and the principal component of flow velocity, which determines the direction of flow.

In aorta, the flow has a helical pattern at the end of systole, in the upper aortic arch as has been described by Kilner [24]; (**Figure 2**) it allows the preservation of laminar flow in the aortic arch. In aortic pathological conditions such as aneurysms, aortic bicuspidi, coarctation, or dissection, rotational flow is abnormal.

6. Three-dimensional printing and virtual reality

Three-dimensional (3D) printing technology has become an attractive tool for creating patient-specific anatomical models (**Figure 3**). Its role in clinical decision and patient management in complex CHD is increasing.

Numerous studies have demonstrated superior advantages of 3D-printed models over the traditional 2D and 3D image reconstructions, enhancing the perception of

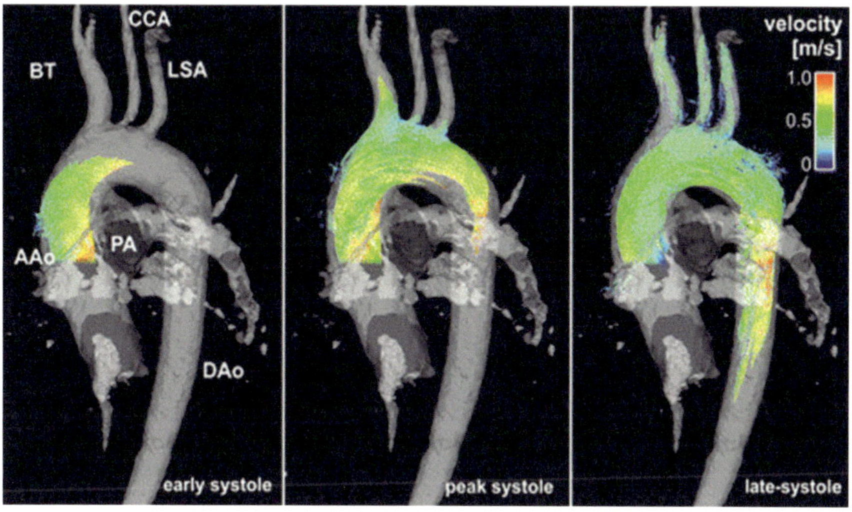

Figure 2.
4D flow CMR of the normal aorta showing the direction of flow in all three phases of systole (early, peak, and end systole).

distances and spatial configuration of the complex cardiac morphology and therefore facilitating the surgical planning [25–27].

A multicenter study [28] showed that the use of 3D-printed heart CHD models enabled surgical decisions to be modified in around 50% of cases.

In a similar way, other studies have confirmed the usefulness of 3D-printed cardiac models to guide surgical procedures in patients with CHD [20, 29–31].

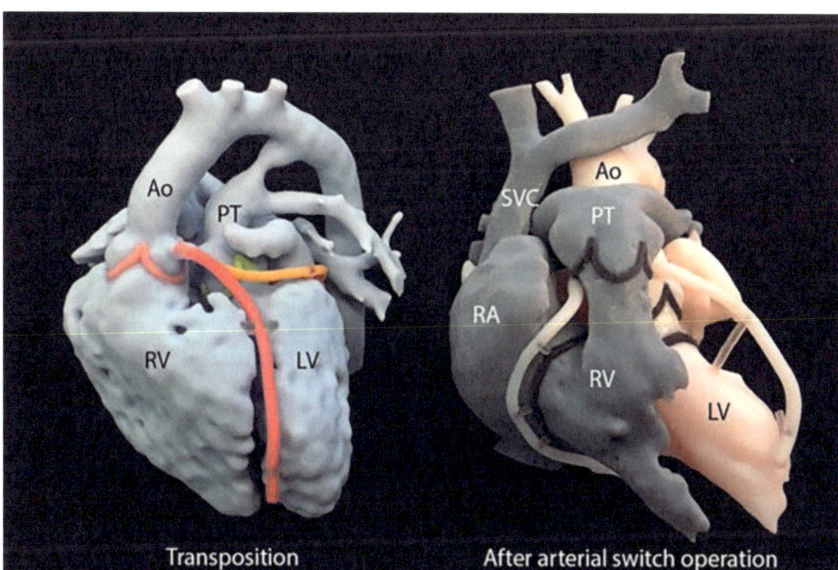

Figure 3.
3D-printed models of transposition of the great arteries and arterial switch operation. Ao, aorta; SVC, superior vena cava; PT, pulmonary trunk; LV, left ventricle; RA, right atrium; RV, right ventricle.

Gomez-Ciriza et al. [32] reported their experience of 7 years in which 3D-printed heart models were able tomodify the surgical decision in 48% of cases.

However, the large application of 3D printing technology in pediatric cardiology practice is still limited by some barriers.

Geographic location: A recent international survey [33] has found that the ability to access 3D printing technology differs from region to region.

The cost of printing materials is another factor that limits its application in many practices, especially soft and elastic materials (high-cost 3D-printed models) with tissue properties similar to normal cardiovascular tissues.

Another limitation of this model is the long time required from image reconstruction to printing and cleaning of the models.

If 3D printing is unavailable, virtual reality (VR) could be a promising technique in clinical application and medical education for CHD. Raimondil and colleagues [34] noticed that the median time to elaborate VR models was only 5 min, which is interesting compared to 3D printing models, which required a long time (8 hours).

7. Interventional CMR

Invasive cardiovascular magnetic resonance imaging (CMR) of cardiac catheterization is a better alternative to fluoroscopy, which has been the gold standard in the assessment of patients with congenital heart disease (CHD). It provides real-time anatomical visualization of the cardiovascular structures [35–37] and the guidance for hemodynamic data without the radiation exposure. The harmful effects of repeated use of X-rays in this population have been increasingly debated in recent years. Prolonged exposure to radiation would be associated with increased risk of cancer in adult patients followed for congenital heart disease [38, 39]. Then, interventional CMR catheterization is a good alternative without ionizing radiation in children, in whom a repetitive hemodynamic assessment would be necessary.

Conditioned catheters and guidewires with gadolinium-filled balloon have been used in CMR-guided cardiac catheterization [40–42].

A few centers reported their experiences with invasive CMR [35, 43–48] for diagnostic and interventional procedures under CMR guidance such as CoA, and Fontan fenestration test occlusion, and pulmonary vein access [49].

ICMR is currently performed in several centers [50], in patients with CHD patients before surgery or in the postoperative follow-up, for diagnostic purposes, in particular catheterization of the right heart in cases of pulmonary hypertension or a more detailed hemodynamic study in complex congenital heart disease (pre-Fontan study, or Fontan fenestration test occlusion, for example,) or for therapeutic purposes (closure of an intercavitary shunt).

The advantage of ICMR is its ability to measure cardiac output and the QP/QS ratio by phase contrast, which have proved to be more reliable than thermodilution, which can be distorted by the presence of a valve leak, or Fick's principle, which gives an estimated rather than measured VO2 value, and at rest rather than during exercise or stress.

In addition, MRI allows ventricular and atrial volumes, EF and functional analysis, and tissue characterization.

Reddy [49] demonstrates the potential of iCMR in diagnostic right and left heart catheterization, CoA diagnosis, and Fontan fenestration occlusion hemodynamic testing.

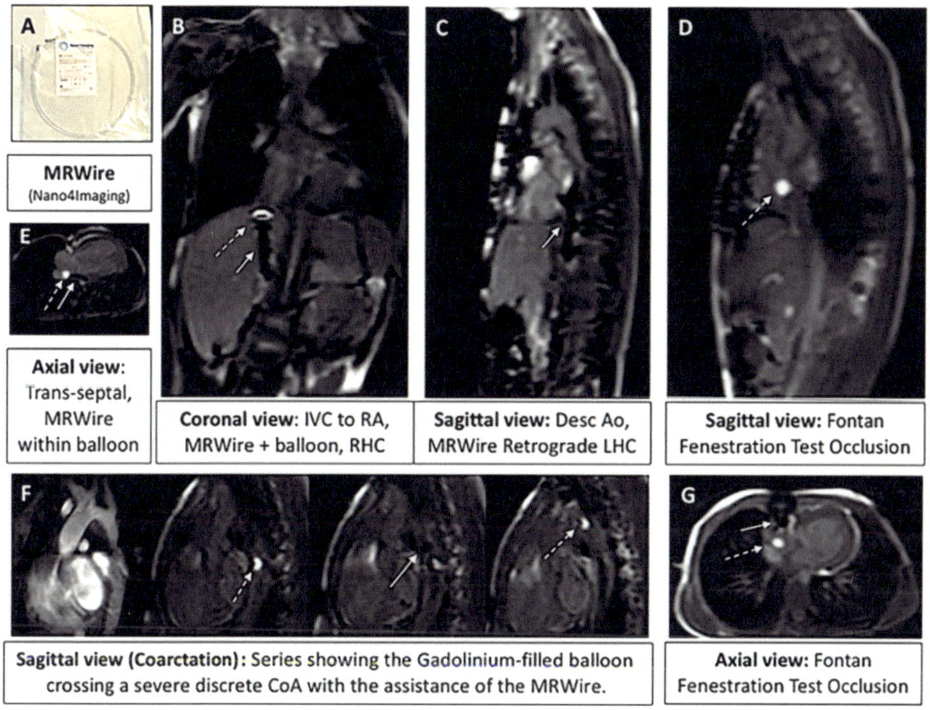

Figure 4.
Series showing a MR-conditional guidewire (a–b solid white arrow) used to guide the gadolinium-filled balloon (dashed white arrow) for a RHC and LHC (c), Fontan fenestration test occlusion, and measure (D–G) of the pulmonary venous saturation in the LA. F: Gadolinium-filled balloon crossing a severe CoA with the assistance of an MR-conditional guidewire. Image courtesy of Surendranath R. Veeram Reddy and Yousef Arar, pediatric cardiology, Children's medical center Dallas, 1935 Medical District Dr., Dallas, TX, 75235, USA.

The balloon attached to the tip of the catheter was filled with diluted gadolinium and guided using a conditioned guide toward the structures to be evaluated hemodynamically, using the real-time sequence (**Figure 4**).

Recently, use of fully insulated nitinol guidewires is feasible in low-SAR and low-field imaging [51, 52].

In the electrophysiology field, CMR allows complete delineation of the atrial anatomy and detection of fibrosis of the left atrium and intra-atrial thrombosis. CMR-guided ablations in particular, cavotricuspid isthmus (CTI) ablation by real-time iCMR guidance is increasingly performed in different centers with similar results to conventional fluoroscopy-guided ablation [53].

8. Conclusion

The new techniques developed over the last decade in cardiac MRI of CHD are promising, offering reduced acquisition and post-processing times while exploring multiple flows in the same examination, thanks to 4D flow, radiation-free diagnostic and therapeutic procedures with ICMR, and accurate anatomical description elaborated by 3D printing in complex CHD. These new tools are currently used in only a few centers and should be accessible in the coming years to the various magnetic resonance imaging centers.

Author details

Karima Hami
Cheikh Zaid Hospital, University Aboulcassis, Rabat, Morocco

*Address all correspondence to: hami7esp@yahoo.com

References

[1] Marelli AJ, Mackie AS, Ionescu-Ittu R, Rahme E, Pilote L. Congenital heart disease in the general population. Circulation. 2007;**115**:163

[2] Bhatt AB, Foster E, Kuehl K, et al. Congenital heart disease in the older adult: A scientific statement from the American Heart Association. Circulation. 2015;**131**(1884-1931):5

[3] Stout KK, Daniels CJ, Aboulhosn JA, et al. 2018 AHA/ACC guideline for the Management of Adults with Congenital Heart Disease: A report of the American College of Cardiology/American Heart Association task force on clinical practice guidelines. Journal of the American College of Cardiology. 2019;**73**:1494-1563

[4] Sachdeva R, Valente AM, Armstrong AK, et al. ACC/AHA/ASE/HRS/ISACHD/SCAI/SCCT/SCMR/SOPE 2020 appropriate use criteria for multimodality imaging during the follow-up care of patients with congenital heart disease. Journal of the American College of Cardiology. 2020;**75**:657-703

[5] Baumgartner H, De Backer J, Babu-Narayan SV, et al. 2020 ESC guidelines for the management of adult congenital heart disease. European Heart Journal. 2021;**42**:563-645

[6] Di Salvo G, Miller O, Babu Narayan S, et al. Imaging the adult with congenital heart disease: A multimodality imaging approach—Position paper from the EACVI. European Heart Journal - Cardiovascular Imaging. 2018;**19**:1077-1098

[7] Sechtem U, Neubauer S, Revel D, De Roos A, Van Rossum A, Von Schulthess G, et al. The clinical role of magnetic resonance in cardiovascular disease. Task force of the European Society of Cardiology, in collaboration with the Association of European Paediatric Cardiologists. European Heart Journal. 1998;**19**:19-39

[8] Friedrich MG. The future of cardiovascular magnetic resonance imaging. European Heart Journal. 2017;**38**:1698-1701

[9] Carlsson M, Töger J, Kanski M, et al. Quantification and visualization of cardiovascular 4D velocity mapping accelerated with parallel imaging or k-t BLAST: Head to head comparison and validation at 1.5 T and 3 T. Journal of Cardiovascular Magnetic Resonance. 2011;**13**:55

[10] Zhong L et al. Intracardiac 4D flow MRI in congenital heart disease: Recommendations on behalf of the ISMRM flow & motion study group. Journal of Magnetic Resonance Imaging. 2019;**50**(3):677-681

[11] Bissell MM et al. 4D CMR Consensus statement 2023 update. Journal of Cardiovascular Magnetic Resonance. 2023;**25**:40

[12] Kamphuis VP, Westenberg JJ, van der Palen RL, et al. Unravelling cardiovascular disease using four dimensional flow cardiovascular magnetic resonance. The International Journal of Cardiovascular Imaging. 2017;**33**(1069-1081):17

[13] Markl M, Wallis W, Harloff A. Reproducibility of flow and wall shear stress analysis using flow-sensitive four-dimensional MRI. Journal of Magnetic Resonance Imaging. 2011;**33**:988-994

[14] Gewillig M. The Fontan circulation. Heart. 2005;**91**:839-846

[15] Hauser JA, Taylor AM, Pandya B. How to image the adult patient with Fontan circulation. Circulation. Cardiovascular Imaging. 2017;**10**:e004273

[16] Puricelli F et al. Performance of cardiac MRI in pediatric and adult patients with Fontan circulation. Radiology Cardiothoracic Imaging. 2022;**4**(3):e210235

[17] Jeong D, Anagnostopoulos PV, Roldan Alzate A, Srinivasan S, Schiebler ML, et al. Ventricular kinetic energy may provide a novel noninvasive way to assess ventricular performance in patients with repaired tetralogy of fallot. The Journal of Thoracic and Cardiovascular Surgery. 2015;**149**:1339-1347

[18] Bokma JP, Geva T, Sleeper LA, Babu Narayan SV, Wald R, et al. A propensity score-adjusted analysis of clinical outcomes after pulmonary valve replacement in tetralogy of Fallot. Heart. 2018;**104**:738-744. DOI: 10.1136/heartjnl-2017-31204

[19] Sjöberg P, Bidhult S, Bock J, Heiberg E, Arheden H, et al. Disturbed left and right ventricular kinetic energy in patients with repaired tetralogy of Fallot: Pathophysiological insights using 4d-flow MRI. European Radiology. 2018;**28**:4066-4076

[20] Fredriksson A, Trzebiatowska-Krzynska A, Dyverfeldt P, Engvall J, Ebbers T, et al. Turbulent kinetic energy in the right ventricle: Potential mr marker for risk stratification of adults with repaired tetralogy of fallot. Journal of Magnetic Resonance Imaging. 2018;**47**:1043-1053

[21] François CJ, Srinivasan S, Schiebler ML, Reeder SB, Niespodzany E, et al. 4D cardiovascular magnetic resonance velocity mapping of alterations of right heart flow patterns and main pulmonary artery hemodynamics in tetralogy of Fallot. Journal of Cardiovascular Magnetic Resonance. 2012;**14**(1):16

[22] Geiger J, Markl M, Jung B, Grohmann J, Stiller B, et al. 4D-mr flow analysis in patients after repair for tetralogy of Fallot. European Radiology. 2011;**21**:1651-1657

[23] Hu L, Ouyang R, Sun A, Wang Q, Guo C, et al. Pulmonary artery hemodynamic assessment of blood flow characteristics in repaired tetralogy of Fallot patients versus healthy child volunteers. Quantitative Imaging in Medicine and Surgery. 2020;**10**:921-933

[24] Kilner PJ, Yang GZ, Mohiaddin RH, Firmin DN, Longmore DB. Helical and retrograde secondary flow patterns in the aortic arch studied by three-directional magnetic resonance velocity mapping. Circulation. 1993;**88**(5 Pt 1):2235-2247

[25] Lau I, Sun Z. Three-dimensional printing in congenital heart disease: A systematic review. Journal of Medical Radiation Sciences. 2018;**65**:226-236. DOI: 10.1002/jmrs.268

[26] Bhatla P, Tretter JT, Chikkabyrappa S, Chakravarti S, Mosca RS. Surgical planning for a complex double-outlet right ventricle using 3D printing. Echocardiography. 2017;**34**:802-804

[27] Biglino G, Milano EG, Capelli C, Wray J, Shearn AI, Caputo M, et al. Three-dimensional printing in congenital heart disease: Considerations on training and clinical implementation from a

teaching session. The International Journal of Artificial Organs. 2019;**42**:595-599

[28] Valverde I, Gomez-Ciriza G, Hussain T, Suarez-Mejias C, Velasco-Forte MN, Byrne N, et al. Three-dimensional printed models for surgical planning of complex congenital heart defects: An international multicentre study. European Journal of Cardio-Thoracic Surgery. 2017;**52**:1139-1148

[29] Kiraly L, Shah NC, Abdullah O, Al-Ketan O, Rowshan R. Three-dimensional virtual and printed prototypes in complex congenital and pediatric cardiac surgery—A multidisciplinary team-learning experience. Biomolecules. 2021;**11**:1703

[30] Cen J, Liufu R, Wen S, Qiu H, Liu X, Chen X, et al. Three-dimensional printing, virtual reality and mixed reality for pulmonary atresia: Early surgical outcomes evaluation. Heart, Lung & Circulation. 2020;**30**:296-302

[31] Ghosh RM, Jolley MA, Mascio CE, Chen JM, Fuller S, Rome JJ, et al. Clinical 3D modeling to guide pediatric cardiothoracic surgery and intervention using 3D printed anatomic models, computer aided design and virtual reality. 3D Printing in Medicine. 2022;**8**:11

[32] Gómez-Ciriza G, Gómez-Cía T, Rivas-González JA, Forte MNV, Valverde I. Affordable three-dimensional printed heart models. Frontiers in Cardiovascular Medicine. 2021;**8**:642011

[33] Illmann CF, Hosking M, Harris KC. Utility and access to 3-dimensional printing in the context of congenital heart disease: An international physician survey study. CJC Open. 2020;**2**:207-213

[34] Raimondi F, Vida V, Godard C, Bertelli F, Reffo E, Boddaert N, et al. Fast-track virtual reality for cardiac imaging in congenital heart disease. Journal of Cardiac Surgery. 2021;**36**:2598-2602

[35] Razavi R, Hill DL, Keevil SF, Miquel ME, Muthurangu V, Hegde S, et al. Cardiac catheterisation guided by MRI in children and adults with congenital heart disease. Lancet. 2003;**362**:1877-1882

[36] Brown DW, Gauvreau K, Powell AJ, Lang P, Colan SD, Del Nido PJ, et al. Cardiac magnetic resonance versus routine cardiac catheterization before bidirectional Glenn anastomosis in infants with functional single ventricle: A prospective randomized trial. Circulation. 2007;**116**:2718-2725

[37] Brown DW, Gauvreau K, Powell AJ, Lang P, del Nido PJ, Odegard KC, et al. Cardiac magnetic resonance versus routine cardiac catheterization before bidirectional Glenn anastomosis: Long-term follow-up of a prospective randomized trial. The Journal of Thoracic and Cardiovascular Surgery. 2013;**146**:1172-1178

[38] Cohen S, Liu M, Gurvitz M, Guo L, Therrien J, Laprise C, et al. Exposure to low-dose ionizing radiation from cardiac procedures and malignancy risk in adults with congenital heart disease. Circulation. 2018;**137**:1334-1345

[39] Roguin A, Goldstein J, Bar O, Goldstein JA. Brain and neck tumors among physicians performing interventional procedures. The American Journal of Cardiology. 2013;**111**:1368-1372

[40] Del Cerro MJ, Moledina S, Haworth SG, Ivy D, Al Dabbagh M,

Banjar H, et al. Cardiac catheterization in children with pulmonary hypertensive vascular disease: Consensus statement from the pulmonary vascular research institute, pediatric and congenital heart disease task forces. Pulmonary Circulation. 2016;**6**(1):118-125

[41] Schmitt B, Steendijk P, Ovroutski S, Lunze K, Rahmanzadeh P, Maarouf N, et al. Pulmonary vascular resistance, collateral flow, and ventricular function in patients with a Fontan circulation at rest and during dobutamine stress. Circulation. Cardiovascular Imaging. 2010;**3**:623-631

[42] Schmitt B, Steendijk P, Lunze K, Ovroutski S, Falkenberg J, Rahmanzadeh P, et al. Integrated assessment of diastolic and systolic ventricular function using diagnostic cardiac magnetic resonance catheterization: Validation in pigs and application in a clinical pilot study. JACC: Cardiovascular Imaging. 2009;**2**:1271-1281

[43] Ratnayaka K, Faranesh AZ, Hansen MS, Stine AM, Halabi M, Barbash IM, et al. Real-time MRI-guided right heart catheterization in adults using passive catheters. European Heart Journal. 2013;**34**:380-389

[44] Pushparajah K, Tzifa A, Bell A, Wong JK, Hussain T, Valverde I, et al. Cardiovascular magnetic resonance catheterization derived pulmonary vascular resistance and medium-term outcomes in congenital heart disease. Journal of Cardiovascular Magnetic Resonance. 2015;**17**:28

[45] Pushparajah K, Tzifa A, Razavi R. Cardiac MRI catheterization: A 10-year single institution experience and review. Interventional Cardiology (London). 2014;**6**:335-346

[46] Rogers T, Ratnayaka K, Lederman RJ. MRI catheterization in cardiopulmonary disease. Chest. 2014;**145**:30-36

[47] Tzifa A, Krombach GA, Kramer N, Kruger S, Schutte A, von Walter M, et al. Magnetic resonance-guided cardiac interventions using magnetic resonance-compatible devices: A preclinical study and first-in-man congenital interventions. Circulation. Cardiovascular Interventions. 2010;**3**:585-592

[48] Tzifa A, Schaeffter T, Razavi R. MR imaging-guided cardiovascular interventions in young children. Magnetic Resonance Imaging Clinics of North America. 2012;**20**:117-128

[49] Surendranath R, Reddy V. Invasive cardiovascular magnetic resonance (iCMR) for diagnostic right and left heart catheterization using an MR-conditional guidewire and passive visualization in congenital heart disease. Journal of Cardiovascular Magnetic Resonance. 2020;**22**:20

[50] Ratnayaka K, Kanter JP, Faranesh AZ, Grant EK, Olivieri LJ, Cross RR, et al. Radiation-free CMR diagnostic heart catheterization in children. Journal of Cardiovascular Magnetic Resonance. 2017;**19**(1):65

[51] Campbell-Washburn AE, Rogers T, Stine AM, Khan JM, Ramasawmy R, Schenke WH, et al. Right heart catheterization using metallic guidewires and low SAR cardiovascular magnetic resonance fluoroscopy at 1.5 tesla: First in human experience. Journal of Cardiovascular Magnetic Resonance. 2018;**20**(1):41

[52] Campbell-Washburn AE, Ramasawmy R, Restivo MC, Bhattacharya I, Basar B, Herzka DA,

et al. Opportunities in interventional and diagnostic imaging by using high-performance low-field-strength MRI. Radiology. 2019;**293**(2):384-393

[53] Rier SC, Vreemann S, Nijhof WH, van Driel V, van der Bilt IAC. Interventional cardiac magnetic resonance imaging: Current applications, technology readiness level, and future perspectives. Therapeutic Advances in Cardiovascular Disease. 2022;**16**:17539447221119624

Section 3

Machine Learning and Brain Network Analysis Methods for MRI

Chapter 4

Applications of Artificial Intelligence in the Classification of Magnetic Resonance Images: Advances and Perspectives

Aron Hernandez-Trinidad, Blanca Olivia Murillo-Ortiz, Rafael Guzman-Cabrera and Teodoro Cordova-Fraga

Abstract

This chapter examines the advances and perspectives of the applications of artificial intelligence (AI) in the classification of magnetic resonance (MR) images. It focuses on the development of AI-based automatic classification models that have achieved competitive results compared to the state-of-the-art. Accurate and efficient classification of MR images is essential for medical diagnosis but can be challenging due to the complexity and variability of the data. AI offers tools and techniques that can effectively address these challenges. The chapter first addresses the fundamentals of artificial intelligence applied to the classification of medical images, including machine learning techniques and convolutional neural networks. Here, recent advances in the use of AI to classify MRI images in various clinical applications, such as brain tumor detection, are explored. Additionally, advantages and challenges associated with implementing AI models in clinical settings are discussed, such as the interpretability of results and integration with existing radiology systems. Prospects for AI in MR image classification are also highlighted, including the combination of multiple imaging modalities and the use of more advanced AI approaches such as reinforcement learning and model generation.

Keywords: artificial intelligence, deep learning, medical imaging, convolutional neural networks, computer-aided diagnosis, automatic classification models

1. Introduction

Medical imaging plays a pivotal role in the diagnosis and treatment of diseases, offering intricate visual insights into the human body [1]. Among the array of available imaging techniques, magnetic resonance imaging (MRI) has witnessed substantial growth in adoption due to its capacity for capturing high-resolution images that exhibit exceptional contrast between soft tissues [2]. The accessibility of magnetic resonance imaging has surged, thanks to advancements in technology and heightened recognition of its clinical value. These images, obtained from various

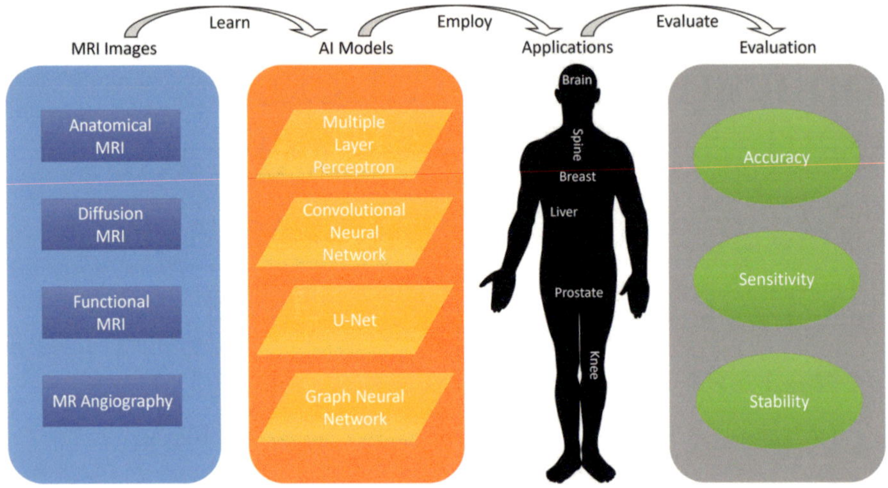

Figure 1.
Organization. We first review MRI images. Next, we introduce common AI models that have been applied to learn those MRI images. Then, we investigate MRI applications that employ AI models. Finally, we discuss the evaluation metrics that are proposed to evaluate how well these AI models are.

anatomical regions and under diverse protocols, furnish indispensable information about anatomical structures, functions, and potential abnormalities [3]. Nevertheless, the interpretation of these MR images presents formidable challenges. Manual analysis by radiologists can be labor-intensive, reliant on expertise, and vulnerable to interobserver variations. Furthermore, the burgeoning volume of images for each patient underscores the imperative for precise and efficient analysis to bolster clinical decision-making [4].

In this context, the application of artificial intelligence (AI) in the classification of magnetic resonance images has emerged as a promising solution [5]. AI holds the potential to process large volumes of images swiftly and accurately, thereby bolstering clinicians in the early detection, characterization, and ongoing monitoring of diseases [6]. Leveraging machine learning techniques and convolutional neural networks, the development of automatic classification models for medical images has demonstrated their competitiveness in comparison to traditional methods [7]. These models excel in discerning subtle patterns and features within MR images, thus facilitating precise diagnoses and prognoses for a myriad of conditions. **Figure 1** illustrates the organization of this chapter.

In summation, given the current landscape of medical imaging with the expanding availability of magnetic resonance images and the compelling need for precise and efficient analysis to underpin clinical decisions, the application of artificial intelligence in image classification is a field of research and development of profound significance [8]. By uniting the computational prowess of AI with the rich, intricate information offered by MR imaging, the potential exists to elevate the accuracy and efficiency of medical diagnosis, ushering in fresh possibilities for patient care.

2. Overview of MRI images

Magnetic Resonance Imaging (MRI) is a non-invasive medical imaging technique that plays a pivotal role in modern healthcare by providing detailed cross-sectional images of the body's internal structures [9]. It operates on the principle of using

DOI: http://dx.doi.org/10.5772/intechopen.113826

strong magnetic fields and radio waves to interact with the hydrogen nuclei (protons) in the body. As these protons align and then return to their natural state within the magnetic field, they emit signals that are captured and processed to generate images. MRI offers various types of images, each with unique applications. T1-weighted images provide excellent anatomical detail, while T2-weighted images are adept at detecting abnormalities like edema and lesions [10]. Proton density (PD)-weighted images emphasize proton concentration, and Diffusion-weighted images (DWI) reveal water molecule movement. Functional MRI (fMRI) maps brain activity, magnetic resonance angiography (MRA) visualizes blood vessels, and magnetic resonance spectroscopy (MRS) assesses tissue chemistry [11]. These images find extensive use in clinical applications, from neuroimaging for brain and spinal conditions to musculoskeletal assessments and cardiovascular evaluations. MRI's advantages include the absence of ionizing radiation, superb soft tissue contrast, and multi-planar imaging capability [12]. However, it can be sensitive to motion artifacts, contraindicated for certain metal implants, and sometimes time-consuming for patients. Nonetheless, MRI remains an invaluable tool, offering detailed insights into the human body's internal structures and functions, thus shaping modern healthcare practices [13]. **Figure 2** illustrates a few examples using different MRI techniques from various human organs.

2.1 Anatomical MRI

One of the fundamental applications of magnetic resonance imaging (MRI) in the realm of medical diagnosis is the visualization of anatomical structures within the human body. Anatomical MRI, often referred to as structural MRI, is a cornerstone of clinical imaging. It provides detailed, high-resolution images of various body parts, offering essential insights into the morphology and integrity of tissues and organs [15].

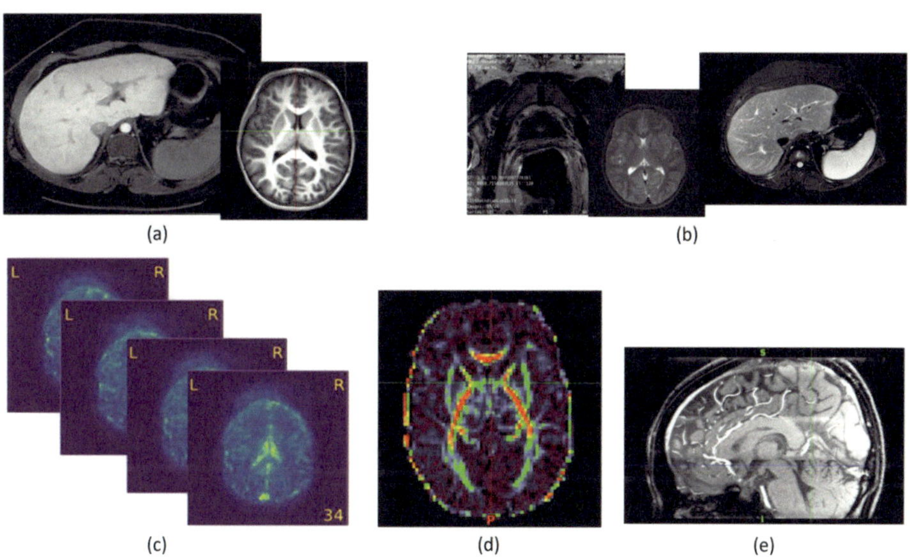

Figure 2.
Illustration of common MRI images. (a) T1-weighted MRI; left: Liver; right: Brain [neonate], (b) T2-weighted MRI; left: Prostate; middle: Brain [neonate]; right: Liver, (c) functional MRI, (d) diffusion tensor imaging, and (e) MR angiography [14].

Anatomical MRI sequences, such as T1-weighted and T2-weighted images, play a crucial role in depicting different tissues based on their inherent physical properties. T1-weighted images offer excellent contrast between fat and water-rich tissues, making them ideal for visualizing anatomical boundaries and structures. In contrast, T2-weighted images highlight variations in water content, effectively revealing abnormalities such as edema, inflammation, or lesions [16].

These MRI sequences are instrumental in diagnosing a wide range of medical conditions. In neuroimaging, they aid in detecting brain abnormalities, such as tumors, vascular malformations, or degenerative diseases like multiple sclerosis. In musculoskeletal imaging, anatomical MRI helps identify soft tissue injuries, joint disorders, and assess the integrity of ligaments and tendons. Additionally, in abdominal imaging, it facilitates the evaluation of organs like the liver, kidneys, and gastrointestinal tract, allowing the detection of tumors, cysts, or structural anomalies.

2.2 Diffusion MRI

Diffusion Magnetic Resonance Imaging (dMRI or diffusion MRI) is a specialized MRI technique that offers a unique window into the microscopic structures and tissue properties within the human body. Unlike traditional anatomical MRI, diffusion MRI focuses on the movement of water molecules within tissues, providing critical information about cellular structures and tissue microarchitecture [17].

At its core, diffusion MRI capitalizes on the inherent Brownian motion of water molecules. In biological tissues, water molecules are not stationary; instead, they exhibit random motion influenced by obstacles such as cell membranes, fibers, and other cellular structures. This random motion, known as diffusion, can be measured, and quantified using diffusion MRI [18].

One of the primary measures derived from diffusion MRI is the apparent diffusion coefficient (ADC), which characterizes the rate and direction of water molecule diffusion within tissues [19]. High ADC values typically indicate free and unrestricted diffusion, often seen in areas with fluid or cystic structures. Conversely, low ADC values suggest restricted diffusion, often associated with dense cellular structures or pathologies that hinder water molecule movement.

Diffusion MRI is particularly valuable in neuroimaging, where it enables the mapping of white matter tracts in the brain. By tracking the diffusion of water molecules along nerve fibers, this technique offers insights into brain connectivity and can identify abnormalities such as white matter lesions, which are common in conditions like multiple sclerosis [20].

2.3 Functional MRI

Functional magnetic resonance imaging (fMRI) is a groundbreaking application of MRI technology that provides real-time insights into the functioning of the human brain. Unlike traditional MRI, which primarily captures structural information, fMRI focuses on the brain's dynamic activity by measuring changes in blood flow and oxygenation levels [21]. At the heart of fMRI lies the concept of neurovascular coupling. When a specific region of the brain becomes active, it requires an increased supply of oxygen and glucose. To meet this demand, blood vessels in the activated area dilate and blood flow surges, leading to an increase in oxygenated hemoglobin levels. This change in blood oxygenation can be detected and visualized by fMRI [22].

Functional MRI is a non-invasive tool that has revolutionized our understanding of brain function and has numerous applications in both clinical and research settings. It enables researchers and clinicians to observe how different brain regions respond to specific tasks, stimuli, or cognitive processes [23]. One of the most prevalent applications of fMRI is functional localization. This technique helps identify critical brain areas responsible for specific functions, such as language processing, motor control, and memory formation. For instance, by instructing a subject to perform language-related tasks during an fMRI scan, researchers can pinpoint the brain regions associated with speech and language functions [24].

In the realm of cognitive neuroscience, fMRI is instrumental in studying complex cognitive processes like decision-making, emotion regulation, and working memory. By examining patterns of brain activation, researchers gain insights into the neural underpinnings of these cognitive functions, paving the way for breakthroughs in fields like psychology and psychiatry [25]. The clinical applications of fMRI are equally profound. It is extensively used in presurgical planning, particularly in cases where brain lesions or tumors are present. fMRI helps surgeons map out functional brain areas, ensuring that critical regions are preserved during surgery to minimize postoperative deficits [26].

2.4 Magnetic resonance angiography (MRA)

Magnetic Resonance Angiography (MRA) is a specialized branch of MRI that focuses on imaging blood vessels, providing detailed visualizations of the vascular system without the need for invasive procedures or contrast agents commonly used in traditional angiography [27]. MRA has evolved as a valuable diagnostic tool in vascular medicine, offering high-resolution images of arteries and veins throughout the body. One of the key advantages of MRA is its non-invasive nature. Unlike conventional angiography, which requires the insertion of catheters and injection of contrast agents, MRA relies solely on the principles of magnetic resonance [28]. Patients undergoing MRA experience no exposure to ionizing radiation or contrast-related risks, making it a safer option, especially for individuals with underlying health conditions.

MRA techniques vary depending on the vascular region of interest, each optimized to provide optimal imaging for specific anatomical areas. Some common MRA techniques include [29]:

- *Time-of-flight (TOF) MRA* [30]: This technique relies on the flow-related enhancement of blood vessels. By utilizing differences in the flow speed of blood, TOF MRA generates high-contrast images of arteries. It is often used for imaging larger vessels, such as the carotid or cerebral arteries.

- *Phase-contrast MRA* [31]: Phase-contrast MRA measures the velocity of blood flow in vessels. By quantifying the phase shifts of moving protons in blood, it produces images that not only visualize vessel anatomy but also provide information about blood flow velocity and direction. This is particularly useful in assessing blood flow dynamics in conditions like stenosis or aneurysms.

- *Contrast-enhanced MRA (CE-MRA)*: In some cases, the use of contrast agents is necessary to enhance the visibility of blood vessels, especially in smaller vessels or when assessing venous structures. CE-MRA involves the injection of a gadolinium-based contrast agent, which shortens the relaxation time of nearby protons, leading to improved vessel visualization.

- *Magnetic resonance venography (MRV)* [32]: MRV is a specific application of MRA tailored to visualize veins. It is commonly used to assess deep vein thrombosis (DVT) in the extremities or to evaluate the venous system in the brain.

The clinical applications of MRA are extensive. It is routinely employed for the diagnosis and evaluation of vascular conditions, including [33]:

- *Atherosclerosis*: MRA can identify narrowing or blockages in arteries caused by atherosclerotic plaques, aiding in the diagnosis of conditions like coronary artery disease and peripheral artery disease.

- *Cerebrovascular disease*: MRA of the brain helps in detecting aneurysms, arteriovenous malformations (AVMs), and other vascular abnormalities that may contribute to strokes or other neurological disorders.

- *Renal artery stenosis*: MRA is a valuable tool for assessing the renal arteries, aiding in the diagnosis of conditions such as renal artery stenosis, which can lead to hypertension and kidney dysfunction.

- *Peripheral vascular disease*: MRA is used to evaluate blood flow in the extremities, assisting in the diagnosis and treatment planning for conditions like deep vein thrombosis (DVT) and peripheral artery disease (PAD).

The integration of artificial intelligence (AI) into MRA analysis holds significant promise. AI algorithms can assist in automating the detection and quantification of vascular abnormalities, improving the efficiency and accuracy of diagnoses. Furthermore, AI-driven predictive models can provide insights into the risk of vascular events and guide personalized treatment strategies [34].

3. Brief introduction of AI models

Artificial Intelligence (AI) has emerged as a transformative force in the field of medical imaging, revolutionizing the way we interpret and utilize various imaging modalities, including Magnetic Resonance Imaging (MRI) [35]. AI models, often powered by deep learning techniques, have demonstrated remarkable capabilities in extracting meaningful information from medical images, thereby aiding in disease diagnosis, treatment planning, and prognosis assessment.

At the heart of AI's impact on medical imaging are neural networks, specifically Convolutional Neural Networks (CNNs) [36]. CNNs have proven highly effective in learning complex patterns and features from images, making them well-suited for tasks such as image classification, segmentation, and object detection. These models mimic the hierarchical organization of neurons in the human brain, enabling them to recognize intricate details within medical images [37]. Two prominent AI models frequently employed in medical imaging are:

- *Convolutional neural networks (CNNs)* [38]: CNNs have become the workhorse of deep learning in medical imaging. They consist of multiple layers of convolutional and pooling operations that systematically extract hierarchical features from images. CNNs excel in tasks like image classification, where they can distinguish between normal and abnormal findings within medical images. Variants of CNNs, such as VGG16, ResNet50, and Inception, have been adapted and fine-tuned for specific medical imaging applications.

- *Recurrent neural networks (RNNs)* [39]: While CNNs dominate image-related tasks, RNNs are specialized for sequential data, making them invaluable for tasks that involve temporal information. In medical imaging, RNNs are particularly useful for processing time-series data, such as functional MRI (fMRI) or dynamic contrast-enhanced MRI (DCE-MRI). They can track changes in image sequences over time, aiding in the assessment of conditions like epilepsy or tumor response to treatment.

AI models in medical imaging go beyond image classification. They are instrumental in tasks like image segmentation, where they identify and outline specific structures or regions of interest within an image. For instance, in MRI, AI can be used to segment tumors, blood vessels, or organs, enabling precise measurements and volumetric assessments [40]. Furthermore, AI models facilitate image registration, aligning images from different modalities or time points, which is crucial for monitoring disease progression or treatment response. They also contribute to generative models, like Generative Adversarial Networks (GANs), which create synthetic medical images for training and augmenting datasets, a particularly useful capability in situations where data is limited [41].

In the realm of AI models for MRI image analysis, a rich tapestry of architectures has emerged, each tailored to specific tasks and challenges. The U-Net architecture, with its intricate encoding and decoding pathways, stands as a stalwart for semantic segmentation tasks, particularly in medical image segmentation [42]. Its ability to capture fine-grained features and preserve spatial information has made it indispensable in delineating anatomical structures. On the other hand, the Multiple Layer Perceptron (MLP) showcases its prowess in handling structured data extracted from MRI images [43]. MLPs are versatile, leveraging dense layers to process information and make predictions, making them suitable for various classification and regression tasks. Meanwhile, Graph Neural Networks (GNNs) have gained traction in MRI analysis by modeling complex relationships within medical data [44]. GNNs excel in tasks requiring the understanding of intricate connections, such as mapping neural pathways or identifying brain regions with functional significance. The adaptability of these architectures further underscores the dynamism of AI models in MRI image analysis, catering to the diverse needs of medical professionals and researchers.

As we delve deeper into this chapter, we will explore the various applications of AI models in the realm of MRI, shedding light on how these models are advancing our ability to extract meaningful insights from medical images. We will discuss their role in image analysis, disease detection, and prognosis assessment, emphasizing their potential to enhance clinical decision-making and patient care. Additionally, we will delve into the latest advancements and future perspectives in AI-driven MRI analysis, highlighting the ongoing research and development in this rapidly evolving field.

4. Deep learning techniques

Deep learning techniques have catalyzed a transformative shift in medical image analysis, propelling the field to new heights in accuracy and efficiency [45]. In the context of Magnetic Resonance Imaging (MRI), these techniques have proven particularly invaluable, enabling the extraction of intricate information from complex images [46]. This section explores the key deep learning techniques employed in MRI analysis, shedding light on their applications and advantages.

4.1 Convolutional neural networks (CNNs)

- *Image classification*: CNNs are the cornerstone of medical image analysis, including MRI. They excel in classifying images into distinct categories, such as normal and abnormal findings or specific disease types. For instance, in brain MRI, CNNs can distinguish between healthy and tumor-affected regions.

- *Segmentation*: CNNs are employed for precise image segmentation, outlining regions of interest within MRI scans. This is crucial for identifying tumors, blood vessels, or anatomical structures. Semantic segmentation, which assigns each pixel in an image to a specific class, is particularly useful in MRI.

4.2 Recurrent neural networks (RNNs)

- *Time-series analysis*: MRI sequences, like functional MRI (fMRI) or diffusion MRI, capture changes over time. RNNs are adept at processing such sequences, enabling the assessment of dynamic processes in the body. For example, fMRI data analysis using RNNs can reveal brain activity patterns related to specific tasks or conditions.

- *Longitudinal studies*: RNNs are indispensable in tracking disease progression or treatment response over multiple MRI scans taken at different time points. They help identify subtle changes that may not be apparent in individual scans.

4.3 Generative adversarial networks (GANs)

- *Data augmentation*: GANs are used to generate synthetic MRI images that closely mimic real data. This aids in data augmentation, increasing the diversity of the training dataset. In MRI, where obtaining labeled data can be challenging, GANs prove invaluable for training robust models.

- *Super-resolution*: GANs are leveraged to enhance MRI image resolution. This is particularly useful in obtaining high-quality images from low-resolution acquisitions, improving the overall diagnostic value.

4.4 Transfer learning

- *Pretrained models*: Transfer learning involves using pretrained deep learning models on large datasets, such as ImageNet, and fine-tuning them for specific MRI analysis tasks [47]. This approach saves computational resources and training time while benefiting from the generalization power of pretrained models.

4.5 Autoencoders

- *Feature extraction*: Autoencoders are utilized for unsupervised feature learning [48]. They compress MRI images into lower-dimensional representations, capturing salient features. These learned features can then be used for various tasks, including classification and segmentation.

4.6 Attention mechanisms

- *Region of Interest (ROI) Attention*: Attention mechanisms enable models to focus on specific regions within an MRI scan [49]. This is particularly useful in cases where only a small part of the image contains diagnostically relevant information. Attention mechanisms help improve model accuracy by emphasizing the important areas.

4.7 3D CNNs

- *Volumetric analysis*: For 3D MRI data, such as volumetric MRI or MRI video sequences, 3D CNNs are employed [50]. These models consider the spatial relationships between image slices, providing a more comprehensive understanding of the 3D structure of anatomical or pathological regions.

4.8 Ensemble models

- *Improved accuracy*: Ensemble models combine predictions from multiple deep learning models, boosting overall accuracy and reducing model variability [51]. In MRI analysis, they are employed to enhance diagnostic reliability and minimize false positives.

4.9 Explainable AI (XAI) techniques

- *Interpretability*: As AI models in MRI analysis become more sophisticated, the need for interpretability grows [52]. XAI techniques, including Grad-CAM and LIME, are applied to elucidate model decisions and provide insights into the features that influence diagnoses.

Deep learning techniques are not only transforming MRI analysis but also pushing the boundaries of what is possible in medical imaging. Their ability to handle complex data, adapt to various modalities, and continuously improve through data-driven learning positions them at the forefront of medical research and clinical applications. In the subsequent sections, we will delve into the specific applications of these techniques in MRI analysis, illustrating their impact on disease detection, prognosis assessment, and treatment planning.

5. AI role in realignment, normalization and registration stages in MRI

The realignment stage in MRI is essential to ensure that the images obtained are of the highest quality possible, especially in clinical applications where patients may move during image acquisition [53]. Here, artificial intelligence has proven to be an invaluable tool in enabling accurate and efficient automation of this process. AI techniques at this stage include:

1. *Landmark tracking*: AI algorithms can identify anatomical landmarks on MRI images, such as prominent bone structures or tissue features. These landmarks are used to track the patient's movements during image acquisition.

2. *Deformation correction*: AI can detect and correct deformations in images caused by patient movement or even magnetic distortions. These corrections are essential to ensure accuracy in applications such as surgical navigation or longitudinal disease assessment.

3. *Real-time image reconstruction*: In situations where real-time motion correction is required, AI can be used to reconstruct images in real-time as they are acquired, correcting any motion instantly.

The use of artificial intelligence in motion realignment and correction not only improves the quality of MRI images, but also reduces the need for repeat studies due to inadvertent patient movements, saving time and resources. Intensity and contrast normalization is crucial to ensure that MRI images are comparable between patients and scanning sessions [54]. Here, artificial intelligence plays an essential role by adjusting image characteristics to facilitate accurate and objective analysis. AI techniques at this stage include:

1. *Normalization standards*: AI algorithms can apply normalization standards to ensure that intensity and contrast in images are consistent across MRI studies. This is especially important when comparing images from different patients or in longitudinal follow-up of the same patient.

2. *Artifact suppression*: AI can identify and suppress artifacts from MRI images, such as those caused by respiratory or metal movements. This significantly improves image quality and diagnostic accuracy.

3. *Improved homogeneity*: AI algorithms can adjust the homogeneity of intensity in images, making it easier to identify subtle structures and pathologies.

Intensity and contrast normalization using artificial intelligence ensures that images are consistent and suitable for clinical interpretation and application of analysis algorithms. Image co-registration in MRI involves aligning multiple sets of images acquired in different sequences or modalities for better comparison and analysis [55]. Artificial intelligence has proven to be highly effective in automating this process. AI techniques at this stage include:

1. *Landmark matching*: AI algorithms can automatically identify anatomical landmarks in different image sets and use them to perform co-registration.

2. *Spatial transformations*: AI can calculate spatial transformations that optimally align images, even when warps or distortions exist.

3. *Multimodal data fusion*: When multiple MRI modalities are used, artificial intelligence can fuse data from different sequences or modalities to provide a more complete and accurate view of anatomy and pathologies.

Image co-registration and data fusion with the help of artificial intelligence are critical for more accurate interpretation and better-informed clinical decision-making in applications involving multiple sets of MRI images.

6. AI applications in MRI

Artificial Intelligence (AI) has revolutionized the field of MRI, offering a plethora of applications that enhance image acquisition, analysis, and clinical decision-making. The fusion of AI and MRI has ushered in a new era of medical imaging, with a wide range of applications that benefit patients and healthcare providers alike [56]. **Table 1** provides a concise overview of how AI enhances various aspects of MRI, from image quality to disease diagnosis and treatment planning.

Application	Description
Image enhancement	Noise reduction: AI reduces noise and artifacts in MRI images. Super-Resolution: AI enhances image resolution for finer anatomical details.
Image reconstruction	Accelerated Imaging: AI-based reconstruction enables faster MRI scans. Sparse Sampling: AI reconstructs high-quality images from sparsely sampled data.
Disease detection and diagnosis	Tumor detection: AI identifies and characterizes tumors in MRI scans. Neurological Disorders: AI aids in diagnosing conditions like Alzheimer's using brain MRI. Cardiovascular diseases: AI assists in detecting heart diseases via cardiac MRI.
Lesion segmentation	AI accurately segments lesions (e.g., tumors) in MRI scans, aiding in treatment planning.
Functional MRI (fMRI) analysis	AI maps brain regions activated during tasks or conditions, facilitating cognitive research.
Diffusion MRI (dMRI) analysis	AI reconstructs white matter tracts in the brain, valuable for neurosurgical planning.
Quantitative imaging	AI quantifies tissue properties (T1, T2, diffusion) for disease characterization. AI analyzes tissue perfusion in MRI, important for diagnosing conditions like stroke.
Automated reporting	AI generates automated radiology reports by extracting findings from MRI scans.
Treatment planning	AI assists in radiotherapy planning by delineating target volumes on MRI.
Monitoring disease progression	AI tracks disease progression by analyzing changes in MRI scans over time.
Predictive modeling	AI predicts disease outcomes and treatment responses based on MRI data.
Quality control	AI performs quality checks on MRI scans, flagging artifacts and anomalies.
Population studies	AI analyzes large MRI datasets for trends, risk factors, and early disease indicators.
Customization and personalization	AI tailors MRI protocols to individual patients for optimized imaging.

Table 1.
Applications of AI in magnetic resonance imaging.

7. AI evaluations in MRI

The evaluation of AI models in the context of MRI images is crucial to assess their performance, accuracy, and clinical utility. One of the fundamental tools for this evaluation is the confusion matrix [57]. The confusion matrix is a table that allows us to visualize the performance of a classification model, particularly in binary classification scenarios, where we are concerned with distinguishing between two classes: positive (disease presence) and negative (disease absence).

7.1 Confusion matrix

The confusion matrix is organized in **Table 2** as follows [58]:
In this confusion matrix:

- *True positives (TP)*: Cases where the AI correctly predicted the presence of a condition.

- *True negatives (TN)*: Cases where the AI correctly predicted the absence of a condition.

- *False positives (FP)*: Cases where the AI incorrectly predicted the presence of a condition when it wasn't there.

- *False negatives (FN)*: Cases where the AI incorrectly predicted the absence of a condition when it was present.

7.2 Key metrics derived from the confusion matrix

Several key metrics can be calculated based on the values in the confusion matrix [59]:

- *Accuracy*: This metric measures the overall correctness of predictions and is calculated as (TP + TN)/(TP + TN + FP + FN). It provides a high-level view of the model's performance but may not be sufficient when dealing with imbalanced datasets.

- *Precision (positive predictive value)*: Precision quantifies the proportion of true positive predictions relative to all positive predictions and is calculated as TP/(TP + FP). It is valuable when minimizing false positives is critical.

- *Recall (sensitivity or true positive rate)*: Recall assesses the model's ability to correctly identify all positive instances and is calculated as TP/(TP + FN). It is crucial when minimizing false negatives is a priority.

	Predicted negative (non-disease)	**Predicted positive (disease)**
Actual negative	True negative (TN)	False positive (FP)
Actual positive	False negative (FN)	True positive (TP)

Table 2.
Confusion matrix for AI model evaluation in MRI images.

- *F1 score*: The F1 score is the harmonic mean of precision and recall and is calculated as 2 * (Precision * Recall)/(Precision + Recall). It provides a balanced evaluation of a model's performance, especially when dealing with imbalanced datasets.

- *Specificity (true negative rate)*: Specificity measures the model's ability to correctly identify all negative instances and is calculated as TN/(TN + FP). It is particularly relevant when the cost of false positives is high.

- *False positive rate (FPR)*: FPR quantifies the proportion of false positives relative to all actual negatives and is calculated as FP/(TN + FP). It is complementary to specificity.

A well-interpreted confusion matrix can provide insights into the strengths and weaknesses of an AI model applied to MRI images. It helps in understanding where the model excels (e.g., high TP and TN) and where it needs improvement (e.g., high FP or FN). Depending on the specific medical application, the choice of evaluation metric may vary. For instance, in cancer detection, high sensitivity (recall) is often prioritized to minimize false negatives, ensuring early disease detection. In contrast, for certain rare conditions, high specificity may be crucial to avoid unnecessary interventions [60].

In addition to traditional evaluation metrics like accuracy, precision, recall, and F1 score, assessing the performance of AI models in MRI image analysis often involves considering other factors such as stability [61]. Stability examines how slight perturbations in the input affect the explanation provided by the model. The stability metric is calculated by dividing the number of stable explanations (those that remain consistent when the input is perturbed) by the total number of explanations generated by the model. A higher stability metric signifies that the AI model's explanations are robust and unaffected by minor variations in the input data. This metric is particularly relevant in medical imaging, where consistency and reliability of model interpretations are paramount. While metrics like stability focus on the model's response to perturbations in the input data, it's important to note that there are various evaluation metrics that do not rely on the confusion matrix but provide valuable insights into the model's performance and behavior [62].

8. Limitations of algorithms in magnetic resonance applications

8.1 Data size and sample requirements

The size of data sets in magnetic resonance imaging (MRI) applications is a critical factor that can influence the effectiveness of machine learning algorithms. Large and diversified data sets are often needed to train high-precision models. However, in practice, it can be difficult to obtain large data sets, which can limit the ability of models to generalize and make accurate diagnoses [63]. In MRI applications, the availability of large data sets may be limited due to various reasons, such as patient privacy or costly and time-consuming data collection. To address these restrictions, data augmentation techniques are used. These strategies involve generating new training samples from existing samples, by applying controlled transformations. Some common forms of data augmentation in MRI include Rotation and Mirroring,

Panning and Zooming, Elastic Distortions, and Noise Aggregation [64]. Transfer learning is another powerful strategy to overcome sample size restrictions in MRI applications. This technique involves leveraging machine learning models pretrained on larger, generic data sets (e.g., models trained on large-scale medical images or even non-medical images) and tailoring them for specific MRI tasks.

8.2 Label quality and annotation challenges

The quality of labels in MRI data sets is essential for training accurate machine learning models. Without accurate and consistent labels, algorithms can produce incorrect or biased results. Data annotation in MRI applications presents several unique challenges due to the detailed and medical nature of the images [65]. Some of these challenges include Expert Requirements, Ambiguity and Variability, Multimodal Data, and Privacy and Security. To address these challenges and improve label quality in MRI applications, several strategies can be employed:

- Formation of scorers
- Consistency and expert agreements
- Cross validation
- Computer aided annotation (CAA) tools
- Quality audit
- Establish a feedback flow
- Active learning

By implementing these strategies, the quality of labels in MRI data sets can be improved, which in turn contributes to training more accurate and reliable machine learning models for medical applications. Furthermore, documentation and monitoring of annotation processes are essential to ensure traceability and data quality.

8.3 Training time and computational resources

The time required to train machine learning models in MRI applications can be significant, especially when complex models are used. This can affect the efficiency of clinical implementation and the ability to respond in critical situations. Training time for AI models in MRI applications can be significant and can vary depending on the complexity of the task and the size of the data set. Some factors that contribute to training time include model architecture, data set size, computational resources, hyperparameters and regularization [66]. Computational resources are critical to accelerate training time and enable efficient deployment of AI models in MRI applications. Some key considerations include graphics processing units (GPU) or tensor processing units (TPU), compute clusters, cloud services, code optimization and transfer learning [67].

Training time and computational resources are critical considerations in AI applications in MRI. Choosing efficient model architectures, optimizing hyperparameters, and accessing high-performance resources are key strategies to reduce training times and improve efficiency in deploying AI models in medical MRI applications.

9. Conclusions

In this chapter, we embarked on a journey through the dynamic intersection of magnetic resonance imaging (MRI) and artificial intelligence (AI). We began by delving into the diverse world of MRI imaging, exploring its various modalities, including anatomical MRI, diffusion MRI, functional MRI (fMRI), and magnetic resonance angiography (MRA). Each modality provided a unique window into the human body, offering invaluable insights for diagnosis and treatment. As we ventured further, we unraveled the power of AI models in revolutionizing MRI image analysis. Deep Learning techniques took center stage, with convolutional neural networks (CNNs) emerging as formidable tools for feature extraction and classification. We explored their versatility across datasets, showcasing their ability to accurately detect a spectrum of medical pathologies.

Applications of AI in MRI proved boundless, from detecting brain tumors in Anatomical MRI to mapping brain activity in fMRI, and even pinpointing vascular anomalies in MRA. Each application underscored the potential to enhance clinical decision-making, optimize resource utilization, and ultimately improve patient outcomes. The evaluation of AI models extended beyond traditional metrics, introducing stability as a crucial factor. We emphasized the importance of robust, consistent model interpretations, especially in the context of medical imaging, where precision is paramount.

In conclusion, the amalgamation of MRI imaging and AI has ushered in a new era of medical diagnostics and patient care. These transformative technologies are poised to reshape the healthcare landscape, offering more accurate, efficient, and reliable tools for medical professionals. With ongoing research, collaboration, and refinement, the future holds the promise of even greater advancements, ultimately benefiting individuals worldwide.

This chapter serves as an overview to the potential of AI in MRI imaging, offering a glimpse into a future where cutting-edge technology and medical expertise converge to improve lives and redefine healthcare standards.

Acknowledgements

We would like to thank the University of Guanajuato and the support of CONAHCyT (scholarship No. 893699).

Conflict of interest

The authors declare no conflict of interest.

Author details

Aron Hernandez-Trinidad[1*], Blanca Olivia Murillo-Ortiz[2], Rafael Guzman-Cabrera[3] and Teodoro Cordova-Fraga[1]

1 Science and Engineering Division, University of Guanajuato Leon Campus, Leon, GTO, Mexico

2 Epidemiology Research Unit IMSS No. 1 High Specialty Medicine Unit, Leon, GTO, Mexico

3 Engineering Division, University of Guanajuato Irapuato-Salamanca Campus, Salamanca, GTO, Mexico

*Address all correspondence to: aron.hernandez@ugto.mx

References

[1] Hill DL et al. Medical image registration. Physics in Medicine & Biology. 2001;**46**(3):R1

[2] Kasban H, El-Bendary MAM, Salama DH. A comparative study of medical imaging techniques. International Journal of Information Science and Intelligent System. 2015;**4**(2):37-58

[3] Lundervold AS, Lundervold A. An overview of deep learning in medical imaging focusing on MRI. Zeitschrift für Medizinische Physik. 2019;**29**(2):102-127

[4] Enzmann DR. Radiology's value chain. Radiology. 2012;**263**(1):243-252

[5] Mazurowski MA et al. Deep learning in radiology: An overview of the concepts and a survey of the state of the art with focus on MRI. Journal of Magnetic Resonance Imaging. 2019;**49**(4):939-954

[6] Gore JC. Artificial intelligence in medical imaging. In: Magnetic Resonance Imaging. Elsevier; 2020. pp. A1-A4

[7] Chattopadhyay A, Maitra M. MRI-based brain tumour image detection using CNN based deep learning method. Neuroscience Informatics. 2022;**2**(4):100060

[8] Adegun AA, Viriri S, Ogundokun RO. Deep learning approach for medical image analysis. Computational Intelligence and Neuroscience. 2021;**2021**:1-9

[9] Liang Z-P, Lauterbur PC. Principles of Magnetic Resonance Imaging. WA: SPIE Optical Engineering Press Belllingham; 2000

[10] Kuperman V. Magnetic Resonance Imaging: Physical Principles and Applications. Elsevier; 2000

[11] Landini L et al. Advanced Image Processing in Magnetic Resonance Imaging. CRC Press; 2018

[12] Katti G, Ara SA, Shireen A. Magnetic resonance imaging (MRI)–a review. International Journal of Dental Clinics. 2011;**3**(1):65-70

[13] Pham TT et al. Magnetic resonance imaging (MRI) guided proton therapy: A review of the clinical challenges, potential benefits and pathway to implementation. Radiotherapy and Oncology. 2022;**170**:37-47

[14] Shamshad F et al. Transformers in medical imaging: A survey. Medical Image Analysis. 2023;**88**:1361-8415

[15] Lenroot RK, Giedd JN. Brain development in children and adolescents: Insights from anatomical magnetic resonance imaging. Neuroscience & Biobehavioral Reviews. 2006;**30**(6):718-729

[16] Durston S et al. Anatomical MRI of the developing human brain: What have we learned? Journal of the American Academy of Child & Adolescent Psychiatry. 2001;**40**(9):1012-1020

[17] Jones DK. Diffusion MRI. Oxford University Press; 2010

[18] Le Bihan D et al. Artifacts and pitfalls in diffusion MRI. Journal of Magnetic Resonance Imaging: An Official Journal of the International Society for Magnetic Resonance in Medicine. 2006;**24**(3):478-488

[19] Sener RN. Diffusion MRI: Apparent diffusion coefficient (ADC) values in the normal brain and a classification of brain disorders based on ADC values.

Computerized Medical Imaging and Graphics. 2001;**25**(4):299-326

[20] Rovaris M et al. Diffusion MRI in multiple sclerosis. Neurology. 2005;**65**(10):1526-1532

[21] Moonen CTW, Bandettini PA. Functional MRI. Vol. 3. Springer; 1999

[22] Van Zijl PCM et al. Quantitative assessment of blood flow, blood volume and blood oxygenation effects in functional magnetic resonance imaging. Nature Medicine. 1998;**4**(2):159-167

[23] DeYoe EA et al. Functional magnetic resonance imaging (FMRI) of the human brain. Journal of Neuroscience Methods. 1994;**54**(2):171-187

[24] Manan HA, Franz EA, Yahya N. Utilization of functional MRI language paradigms for pre-operative mapping: A systematic review. Neuroradiology. 2020;**62**:353-367

[25] Szaflarski JP et al. Comprehensive presurgical functional MRI language evaluation in adult patients with epilepsy. Epilepsy & Behavior. 2008;**12**(1):74-83

[26] Park KY et al. Mapping language function with task-based vs. resting-state functional MRI. PLoS One. 2020;**15**(7):e0236423

[27] Dumoulin CL, Hart HR Jr. Magnetic resonance angiography. Radiology. 1986;**161**(3):717-720

[28] Hartung MP, Grist TM, François CJ. Magnetic resonance angiography: Current status and future directions. Journal of Cardiovascular Magnetic Resonance. 2011;**13**(1):1-11

[29] Potchen EJ. Magnetic Resonance Angiography: Techniques, Indications and Practical Applications. Springer; 2006

[30] Laub GA. Time-of-flight method of MR angiography. Magnetic Resonance Imaging Clinics of North America. 1995;**3**(3):391-398

[31] Dumoulin CL. Phase contrast MR angiography techniques. Magnetic Resonance Imaging Clinics of North America. 1995;**3**(3):399-411

[32] Carpenter JP et al. Magnetic resonance venography for the detection of deep venous thrombosis: Comparison with contrast venography and duplex Doppler ultrasonography. Journal of Vascular Surgery. 1993;**18**(5):734-741

[33] Carr JC, Carroll TJ. Magnetic Resonance Angiography: Principles and Applications. Springer Science & Business Media; 2011

[34] Yasaka K et al. Impact of deep learning reconstruction on intracranial 1.5 T magnetic resonance angiography. Japanese journal of. Radiology. 2022;**40**(5):476-483

[35] Huang S-C et al. Developing medical imaging AI for emerging infectious diseases. Nature Communications. 2022;**13**(1):7060

[36] Li Z et al. A survey of convolutional neural networks: Analysis, applications, and prospects. IEEE Transactions on Neural Networks and Learning Systems. 2021;**33**:2162-237X

[37] Wu J. Introduction to convolutional neural networks. National Key Lab for Novel Software Technology. Nanjing University. China. 2017;**5**(23):495

[38] Albawi S, Mohammed TA, Al-Zawi S. Understanding of a Convolutional Neural Network. IEEE; 2017

[39] Medsker LR, Jain LC. Recurrent neural networks. Design and Applications. 2001;**5**(64-67):2

[40] Pereira S et al. Brain tumor segmentation using convolutional neural networks in MRI images. IEEE Transactions on Medical Imaging. 2016;**35**(5):1240-1251

[41] Creswell A et al. Generative adversarial networks: An overview. IEEE Signal Processing Magazine. 2018;**35**(1):53-65

[42] Yin X-X et al. U-net-based medical image segmentation. Journal of Healthcare Engineering. 2022;**2022**:1-16

[43] Singh J, Banerjee R. A Study on Single and Multi-Layer Perceptron Neural Network. IEEE; 2019

[44] Wu Z et al. A comprehensive survey on graph neural networks. IEEE Transactions on Neural Networks and Learning Systems. 2020;**32**(1):4-24

[45] LeCun Y, Bengio Y, Hinton G. Deep learning. Nature. 2015;**521**(7553): 436-444

[46] Liu J et al. Applications of deep learning to MRI images: A survey. Big Data Mining and Analytics. 2018;**1**(1):1-18

[47] Weiss K, Khoshgoftaar TM, Wang D. A survey of transfer learning. Journal of Big Data. 2016;**3**(1):1-40

[48] Tschannen M, Bachem OF, Lučić M. Recent advances in autoencoder-based representation learning. In: Bayesian Deep Learning Workshop, NeurIPS. 2018. 47658

[49] Niu Z, Zhong G, Yu H. A review on the attention mechanism of deep learning. Neurocomputing. 2021;**452**:48-62

[50] Klaiber M et al. A Systematic Literature Review on Transfer Learning for 3d-CNNs. IEEE; 2021

[51] Sagi O, Rokach L. Ensemble learning: A survey. Wiley Interdisciplinary Reviews: Data Mining and Knowledge Discovery. 2018;**8**(4):e1249

[52] Gunning D et al. XAI—Explainable artificial intelligence. Science Robotics. 2019;**4**(37):eaay7120

[53] Mathiak K, Posse S. Evaluation of motion and realignment for functional magnetic resonance imaging in real time. Magnetic Resonance in Medicine: An Official Journal of the International Society for Magnetic Resonance in Medicine. 2001;**45**(1):167-171

[54] Shah M et al. Evaluating intensity normalization on MRIs of human brain with multiple sclerosis. Medical Image Analysis. 2011;**15**(2):267-282

[55] Stefano A et al. Robustness of pet radiomics features: Impact of co-registration with mri. Applied Sciences. 2021;**11**(21):10170

[56] Turkbey B, Haider MA. Deep learning-based artificial intelligence applications in prostate MRI: Brief summary. The British Journal of Radiology. 2022;**95**(1131):20210563

[57] Visa S et al. Confusion matrix-based feature selection. Maics. 2011;7**10**(1):120-127

[58] Krstinić D et al. Multi-label classifier performance evaluation with confusion matrix. Computer Science & Information Technology. 2020;**1**:1-14

[59] Hossin M, Sulaiman MN. A review on evaluation metrics for data classification evaluations. International Journal of Data Mining & Knowledge Management Process. 2015;**5**(2):1

[60] Dalianis H, Dalianis H. Evaluation metrics and evaluation. In: Clinical Text Mining: Secondary Use of Electronic Patient Records. 2018. pp. 45-53

[61] Prabhu AM, Choksi TS. Data-driven methods to predict the stability metrics of catalytic nanoparticles. Current Opinion in Chemical Engineering. 2022;**36**:100797

[62] Farahani FV et al. Explainable AI: A review of applications to neuroimaging data. Frontiers in Neuroscience. 2022;**16**:906290

[63] McCradden MD et al. Ethical limitations of algorithmic fairness solutions in health care machine learning. The Lancet Digital Health. 2020;**2**(5):e221-e223

[64] Chlap P et al. A review of medical image data augmentation techniques for deep learning applications. Journal of Medical Imaging and Radiation Oncology. 2021;**65**(5):545-563

[65] Monarch RM. Human-in-the-Loop Machine Learning: Active Learning and Annotation for Human-Centered AI. Simon and Schuster; 2021

[66] Grolinger K, Capretz MAM, Seewald L. Energy Consumption Prediction with Big Data: Balancing Prediction Accuracy and Computational Resources. IEEE; 2016

[67] Chen C et al. Deep learning on computational-resource-limited platforms: A survey. Mobile Information Systems. 2020;**2020**:1-19

Chapter 5

Resting-State fMRI Advances for Functional Brain Dynamics

Denis Larrivee

Abstract

The development of functional magnetic resonance imaging (fMRI) in quiescent brain imaging has revealed that even at rest, brain activity is highly structured, with voxel-to-voxel comparisons consistently demonstrating a suite of resting-state networks (RSNs). Since its initial use, resting-state fMRI (RS-fMRI) has undergone a renaissance in methodological and interpretive advances that have expanded this functional connectivity understanding of brain RSNs. RS-fMRI has benefitted from the technical developments in MRI such as parallel imaging, high-strength magnetic fields, and big data handling capacity, which have enhanced data acquisition speed, spatial resolution, and whole-brain data retrieval, respectively. It has also benefitted from analytical approaches that have yielded insight into RSN causal connectivity and topological features, now being applied to normal and disease states. Increasingly, these new interpretive methods seek to advance understanding of dynamic network changes that give rise to whole brain states and behavior. This review explores the technical outgrowth of RS-fMRI from fMRI and the use of these technical advances to underwrite the current analytical evolution directed toward understanding the role of RSN dynamics in brain functioning.

Keywords: resting-state networks, resting-state fMRI, big data analysis, high strength magnetic imaging, effective connectivity, parallel imaging, independent components analysis

1. Introduction

Resting-state, functional, magnetic resonance imaging (RS-fMRI) focuses on spontaneous low-frequency fluctuations (< 0.1 Hz) in the BOLD signal that occur in the absence of task-related activities. The functional significance of these fluctuations was first recognized by Biswal et al. [1] in a study in which subjects were told not to perform any cognitive, language, or motor tasks. After determining the correlation between the BOLD time course of a seed region identified by bilateral finger tapping and that of all other areas in the brain, the authors found that fluctuations in the left somatosensory cortex were highly correlated with homologous areas in the contralateral hemisphere. This observed correlation led to their conclusion that such "resting networks" manifested the functional connectivity of the brain.

The observation of spontaneous, synchronous fluctuations occurring between brain regions has since stimulated studies that have identified as many as 7 to 17 other stable networks [2–5], although seven are consistently agreed upon. The visual network, for example, is highly consistent across various studies and spans much of the occipital cortex. The importance of this network structure is reflected in the amount of bodily energy devoted toward brain and, presumably, network maintenance. On a relative basis, the energy consumed by the brain is approximately 20% of the total bodily energy consumption, despite a relative mass of only 2%. Of the brain's consumption, some 60 to 80% of the energy is used while "resting," which is for internal communication and support alone. By contrast, elicited activity consumes less than 1% of the brain's energy resources. Resting networks thus appear to constitute a fundamental organizational architecture for the functional properties of the brain [5].

Because characterization of resting-state networks (RSNs) in the human brain relies on the analysis of temporal fluctuations in the blood oxygenation level-dependent (BOLD) signal, the delineation of RSNs has been directly linked to the ability of fMRI to detect neural activity [6]. Using T2-weighted signal intensity and blood oxygenation as the contrast agent [7], fMRI imaging offers a relatively facile procedure for the acquisition of brain activity data [8, 9], one that has been exploited in numerous studies.

Early investigations [10] confirmed fMRI suitability for RSN determinations. The advantages of RS-fMRI in its own right have since become apparent [8], including ease of signal acquisition, minimal requisite effort from the patients, and proficiency for identifying functional areas in different patient populations. Recent studies have demonstrated that imaging of difficult-to-monitor patients, such as pediatric subjects and patients with disorders of consciousness, that is, coma, vegetative, and minimally conscious states, are able to undergo RS-fMRI. The procedure also offers the capability for functional differentiation, when patients perform specific tasks that are designed to target a single network such as motor, language, memory, vision, attention, and sensory networks.

Despite limitations in use of the BOLD signal, especially the dichotomy between the temporal resolution and the temporal scale of the neural activity measured, RS-fMRI studies have continued to expand, propelled not only by technical improvements at the level of signal acquisition—e.g., parallel MRI imaging, data acquisition [11], and computational advances for preprocessing and feature extraction [12]—but also by theoretical and mathematical tools that have amplified the functional interpretations of quiescent and task-based brain activity [13, 14]. One outcome of these developments has been a more precise view of how RSNs are functionally organized and how this in turn modulates communication within the brain, that is, a more dynamic view of information exchange and regulation [15].

The need to address cognitive dysfunction in the light of these more precise and advanced models of brain operation has also benefitted from this work. The DMN has been an early and continuing focus of study for the exploration of alterations during Alzheimer's and other degenerative diseases, which tend to adapt to the structural profile of the network [16]. There is also increasing interest in examining the neurological changes that occur as a result of traumatic, vascular, or oncological influences, which, because of their focal impact, can affect multiple network domains [17, 18]. Stroke, especially, is a leading cause of disability and dependency in adults—in 2010, there were about 11.6 million incident ischemic stroke events in the United States, and by 2030, an additional 3.4 million adults are predicted to have strokes.

In light of RSN discoveries, the understanding of how these focal effects influence brain functioning has also evolved. Stroke lesions are therefore understood not only to result in focal, location-dependent neurological symptoms but can also induce widespread effects in remote regions in the affected and unaffected hemispheres. Consistent with this, while baseline measures of stroke severity represent the current level of diagnostic and prognostic capability, patients' neurological impairment sometimes exceeds what would be expected from stroke magnitude; that is, growing evidence emphasizes the role of distributed neural networks in the generation of brain states and the control of behavior that could account for stroke outcomes affecting behavior [18, 19]. Such possibilities implicate a need for still more comprehensive RSN tools that can explore the relationship between whole-scale RSN dynamics and behavior in clinical settings.

This review discusses the evolution in the study of brain RSNs as an outgrowth of the methodological principles that have advanced fMRI imaging of neural brain activity. It covers the advances in technical approaches for data retrieval and processing that have provided the basis for improved network analysis and that build on conceptual insights into functional network associations based on connectivity associations. It also considers both the frequently used data-driven approaches and their contribution to larger-scale explorations of brain dynamics based on causal connectivities and topological variation, now being applied in more global models. Improvements in these latter are likely to offer the prospect of clinical insights that can relate network operation to disease states, such as stroke.

2. Modern resting state network methodology

2.1 Resting-state network detection as an outgrowth fMRI

RS-fMRI relies on spontaneous low-frequency fluctuations (< 0.1 Hz) in the BOLD signal, which measures the contrast between the diamagnetic effect of oxy-hemoglobin and the paramagnetic effect of deoxy-hemoglobin [7]. The dependence on the BOLD signal means that RS-fMRI shares advantages that accrue to fMRI—the ability to monitor neural activity, albeit indirectly—but also disadvantages that characterize its use. Chief among these limitations is fMRI's temporal resolution, which is dependent on the hemodynamic response time. Since the hemodynamic response is much slower than the underlying neural processes, temporal information of spiking events is heavily blurred and typically requires the use of mathematical processing, like that of the general linear model [9], or experimental block protocols, to infer event-related, signal activity. With processing, temporal resolution in the 100 ms range can be achieved, which is roughly tenfold slower than the neural events being monitored. By contrast, the spatial resolution of fMRI is considerably better, as well as much superior to electrical and magnetic recording techniques, though slightly reduced from that of MRI. Due to the need for fast acquisition of time series information, the spatial resolution in the case of fMRI is limited somewhat by the signal-to-noise ratio (SNR). With single-shot imaging, for example, the acquisition time for fMRI is reduced and the pixel size must be increased to obtain a satisfactory SNR. With a suitable increase in magnetic strength [20], however, SNR is sufficiently enhanced to yield a pixel size slightly under 1 mm.

A key factor in the use of RS-fMRI is the measurement of neural activity fluctuations rather than spiking events per se. Neural activity fluctuations (low-frequency and indirectly measured using the BOLD signal) exhibit substantially different time courses from those of neural firing (high-frequency and direct). Accordingly, while the representation of individual, high-frequency spiking events is itself heavily blurred, the slow neural activity fluctuations detected by the BOLD signal display a well-resolved temporal pattern. Measurements of these fluctuations thus provide for accurate functional inferences obtained from voxel-to-voxel comparisons. Together with the high spatial resolution that is an inherent feature of fMRI, RS-fMRI currently constitutes the most powerful tool available for assessing the functional connectivity properties of brain networks.

2.2 Technical advances in RS-fMRI

2.2.1 General acquisition

The early detection of RSNs by Biswal et al. [10] used a standard 1.5 T clinical scanner equipped with a three-axis head gradient coil and a shielded birdcage radio frequency coil. A time course of 512 echo-planar images (EPI) from a 10 mm axial slice (flip angle 34°) was obtained every 250 ms and the respective data sets were band pass filtered at <0.08 Hz. Using these moderate parameters, the study demonstrated a high degree of temporal correlation in the sensorimotor cortex and in several other regions associated with motor function. Departing from this early protocol, most RS-fMRI scanning now employs 3 Tesla (3 T) field strength to obtain clinically reliable data and gradient-echo echo-planar imaging (GE-EPI) sequences [21, 22]. Because RSN acquisition is T2* weighted, GE sequencing is typically used in preference to T2 weighted spin echo sequences [23]. Whole-brain coverage is required, with high in-plane resolution (about 2 to 3 mm) and a repeat time (TR) of 2 to 3 s [24] to capture the distributed configuration of RSNs.

While most RS-fMRI imaging studies rely on these or comparable protocols, current resting-state procedures also have available an arsenal of advances that can supplement the current standard conditions. Among other developments, these include procedures for increasing data acquisition speed [22], enhancing spatial resolution by improving SNR capabilities with high-strength magnetic fields [20], preprocessing corrections for motion artifacts [25], and big data acquisition capability [26].

2.2.2 Rapid data acquisition

The advent of parallel imaging has stimulated an increasing number of studies that have sought to harness the speed of data acquisition made possible by its development [11]. Fast RS-fMRI has been motivated by various objectives. Firstly, increasing data acquisition speed can assist multivariate approaches while also retaining a comparable level of sensitivity. For clinical groups for whom RS-fMRI is an increasingly used diagnostic approach, this affords greater interpretive power [27]. The use of rapid data approaches also enables better discretization of dynamical changes associated with connectivity changes, which are posited to reflect distinct brain states [28–30]. Additionally, rapid RS-fMRI data acquisition can help to identify artifactual contributions, such as cardiac and respiratory rhythms [31, 32]. With low sampling rates, these sources of physiological noise often alias to lower, functionally associated, frequency bands [33] making them difficult to resolve since task time series are unavailable in the resting state [34].

Parallel MRI imaging employs multiple receiver coils for fast data acquisition. These capture spatially distinct data sets due to the differential spatial profiles of the receivers. The most widely used configurations are Multiband (MB) and 3D echo planar imaging (EPI) [35]. Multiband pulses excite a set number of slices simultaneously, ranging from MB2–4 up to MB8, which are then unfolded. Faster sampling rates can be achieved by reducing the overlap between slices with techniques like GRAPPA or CAIPIRINHA [36–39]. Both of these techniques operate in the frequency domain and are based on the principle that k space information within a given point is partially retained in neighboring points of the k domain, which can be retrieved during scanning. The CAIPIRINHA technique is an evolution of the GRAPPA technique, in which there is an applied acceleration along the K_y and K_z directions and an additional phase offset (slice-shift) along the K_z direction. These modifications yield unique frequency patterns and therefore simpler aliasing to solve. In 3D EPI, the slice direction is embedded with a phase encoding gradient. Each repetition excites the whole imaging volume, requiring a smaller flip angle. The use of the encoding gradient also accelerates data acquisition, which when used in conjunction with the CAIPIRINHA approach, can still achieve faster retrieval [40].

Another approach used for rapid data retrieval is that of Magnetic Resonance Electroencephalography (MREG). This approach derives its speed from the ability to traverse the k-space with a stack of spiral trajectories [41], which significantly reduces sampling recovery, enabling whole data scans in less than 100 ms. A drawback is the relatively low spatial resolution of about 3 mm. However, the method offers the significant advantage of greatly facilitating dynamic functional connectivity analyses [42] that require large data sets.

2.2.3 High strength fields in RS-fMRI

Although most RS-fMRI studies are conducted at 3 T, higher field strengths offer advantages not provided by standard 3 T field strength. Higher field strengths yield correlation coefficients that are consistently higher for resting networks, due to the linear dependency of the SNR on the magnetic field [43, 44]. The higher correlation and enhanced signal combine to improve signal detection and lessen the amount of mathematical processing needed for signal resolution, which means that the spatial characteristics of resting networks can be measured with greater precision than at lower field strengths. The chief advantage of higher fields thus is an improved spatial resolution, which enables a better spatial delineation of network maps.

Additionally, due to the higher SNR, the temporal reliability of mapping is also improved, lending the technique a broader clinical range. For example, RS-fMRI at 7 T has been shown to enhance the temporal reliability of sensorimotor and language network detection in preoperative planning [45] and for mapping habenula resting-state networks involved in anxiety and addiction disorders [46].

On the other hand, use of higher field strengths has several drawbacks, including longer sampling intervals, inhomogenous magnetic field properties, and the logarithmic growth in specific absorption rate (SAR) with increasing field strength [22]. In particular, the higher spatial resolution requires long repetition times, due to the need to include data acquisition from the whole brain to accommodate the brain-wide distribution of major RSNs. Additionally, inhomogeneities in magnetic field affect receive and transmit RF coil sensitivity [47], which requires correction for accurate connective mapping, while SAR constraints on echo planar imaging affect multiband pulses [22].

2.2.4 Big data

Current increases in study size are generating exceptional amounts of data in their attempts to explore ever-larger studies of RSNs in brain operation. The Human Connectome Project [48] and the 1000 Functional Connectomes Project [49] have released in excess of 1000 RS-fMRI data sets, for example. Traditional data-driven methods for handling RS-fMRI data, such as independent components analysis and graph theoretic approaches, become unwieldy and lose descriptive power at elevated data levels. The need for suitable techniques to address big data handling is thus currently stimulating the development of new preprocessing methods and analytical adaptions that can accurately reflect network structure and dynamics [50].

Large data sets are typically characterized in three ways, the amount of data, termed Big Volume, the diversity of information, termed Big Variety, and the reliability of the data as a representation of brain functional architecture, termed Big Veracity. Big-volume RSN data sets are characterized by an informational mass exceeding that of a single very large computer processing capacity [50], though not so large as whole genome data sets. Big variety reflects the diversity of information within a single data set but can also extend to comparisons between two data sets, such as occurs with two or more imaging data sets or with other information modes like behavior, for example, the Open Access Series of Imaging Studies (OASIS) project with more than 500 subjects worth of data [51]. Big Veracity considers the various data sources that can lessen the ability to extract meaningful network data, including noise, resolution artifacts, data inconsistencies, and acquisition errors.

Initial steps involved in big data handling entail preprocessing to remove the effects of sources that diminish the ability to assess meaningful data. Several preprocessing steps are becoming more accepted, but these can also greatly increase computational load. The most widely used is the minimal preprocessing pipeline [50]. Its goal is to provide RS-fMRI data for analysis with a minimum level of quality, which also minimizes the loss of meaningful data. This can be of substantial benefit to researchers lacking access to high-powered preprocessing of Big Volume data sets. Currently, preprocessing software tools tend to adopt a parallelization approach with functions running in parallel for tools such as statistical parametric mapping (SPM) [50].

Analytical procedures have tended to emphasize graph-theoretic tools that are amenable to statistical mechanical methods. One of the most used topological tools is Mapper, developed by Singh et al. [52], which adopts a persistent homology approach. Mapper lends itself to big data analysis because the global organizational structure is divided into a series of overlapping slices. These are reconstructed *via* the use of common points located in the overlapping zones, which serve as a vehicle to orient topology.

3. Assessing functional connectivity in RSN data

Several approaches have been developed to analyze imaging data after preprocessing and band-pass filtering. These include approaches driven by research focus as well as those dictated by the data itself, the so-called data-driven and model-free approaches. Each can be used to delineate the distribution of functional connections that characterize major networks of the brain.

3.1 Regions of interest seed-based analyses

Functional connectivity determinations extend fMRI measurements of brain activity by providing likelihood estimates of functional associations between neural activity zones [1]. In practice, seed-based analyses identify deviations from independence between distributed and often distant sources of neural activity and a region of interest; that is, statistically significant deviations from independence reveal dependent relationships that functionally connect activity zones. Extending these relationships to multiple zones enables the construction of connectivity maps that become identified with unique networks. Exploiting a seed-based ROI strategy, for instance, one comprehensive study of resting-state fMRI sequences from 1000 healthy adults [53] revealed seven functionally connected networks at coarse resolution and 17 at fine resolution. The simplicity and interpretability of the ROI technique make it procedurally facile and a frequently adopted approach. However, the method relies entirely on user-defined ROIs and so is limited for network discovery by its a priori, selected criteria.

3.2 Independent components analysis (ICA)

In light of this caveat, coupled with the evolution of mathematical models and improved computational capabilities, there has been a paradigm shift from that of imposing initial conditions, that is, seed-based ROIs, on the data to that of extracting patterns of brain activity directly from the raw time series. The main example of this approach is independent components analysis. In this approach, the time series signal is assumed to be due to multiple spatio-temporal processes that are statistically independent of each other. By extracting the independent signals, various time courses of specific brain regions can be constructed and grouped into maps representative of their spatial distribution.

Independent components analysis (ICA) aims at overcoming the selective bias toward priors contained in seed-based approaches by relying on direct data-driven interrogation for assessment of functional connectivity [54]. To do so, ICA posits an inherent representation of independent factors in the captured time series data. Its goal is to decompose the vector representation of these factors, Z, as a product of a combinatorial matrix and the spatially independent components where:

$$Z = NC + E = \sum_{j=1}^{J} n_j c_j + E, \quad (1)$$

Here, N is a $T \times J$ combinatorial matrix with columns n_j, and C is the $J \times Nv$ matrix of independent components with rows c_j, where each c_j corresponds to component j for a cumulative total of J independent components. These components represent the networks of various functions. The elements of the matrix E are independent, normally distributed noise contributions. It is presumed that the component maps, $c_j, j = 1, \ldots, J$ contain overlapping and statistically dependent signals, but that the individual component map distributions are independent. Each independent component c_j is a vector of size Nv and represents the relative amount of a given voxel that is modulated by the activation of that component. Due to the retrieval of large data during the acquisition stage, various algorithms have been developed to estimate the components, for example, the independent components analysis with a reconstruction cost (RICA) algorithm [55].

3.3 Graph theory analysis

Another approach to the interpretation of RS-fMRI datasets employs graph theory, where activity sources comprise nodes and connectivity defines the edges that link these nodes [56]. Unlike ICA, which focuses chiefly on the strength of correlation between different domains, graph theory characterizes the features of network topology. The graph theory approach describes the interaction between nodes by means of such graph parameters as average path length, clustering coefficients, node degree, centrality measures, and level of modularity. Graph theory is thus a promising technique for exploring the integration and segregation of networks in the brain. Graph metrics like average path length, for example, reveal the extent of integration of brain networks. Centrality, on the other hand, examines whether a particular node has a central or leading role in information segregation *via* its propagation to other nodes in a network.

Increasingly, modularity assessments have been used to characterize functional adjustments occurring during behavior, network perturbations, or pathologies that affect network function and the observed values have been shown to undergo significant alteration in such pathologies as stroke [57] and psychiatric disease [58–60]. Modularity assesses the presence of functionally independent units or modules that compose resting-state networks. These are defined as clusters of nodes displaying greater functional connectivity within the group than with the rest of the brain. During task-specific activity, such clusters are reallocated, implying that the networks themselves are reorganized topologically [61, 62]. Their flexibility suggests that they operate as independent functional entities inducing [63–65] specific behaviors *via* their reallocation [66, 67].

In practice, modularity analysis [63] describes the difference between the network configuration at rest and the network reconfiguration during behaviorally altered conditions by means of a quality function (Q) [68] that maximizes the optimal modular decomposition. As expressed by Q, the modularity index provides a measure of the degree of modular segregation [69], where Q is close to one when there are few edges between modules and high density inside modules—that is, module segregation is present—and Q is close to zero when the number of connections between modules is comparable to that of random—indicating an absence of segregation.

3.4 RSN functional connectivity maps

The first demonstration of correlated spontaneous fluctuations explored somatosensory areas. Since this initial demonstration, multiple other resting networks have been discovered. Functional connectivity determinations have shown that these networks can be reliably reproduced [53], although much variation in the identification of networks is dependent on the degree of resolution achieved during scanning. Major resting networks, according to Yeo's seven network parcellation atlas [4, 53], are listed in **Table 1** and classed broadly as belonging to either sensorimotor or association groups. While numerically greater numbers of networks can be detected at finer resolution, e.g., 17 network estimate of Yeo et al. [53], generally, the 17-network determination fractionates the lesser member set into smaller network components of the seven major networks.

Network	Type	Description
Default Mode Network a	Association	Contains the dorsal prefrontal cortex, posterior cingulate cortex, precuneus, and angular gyrus
Dorsal Attention Network. n s	Association	Includes gyri adjacent to the intraparietal sulcus, cortex near the MT + complex, and both the frontal and secondary eye-fields
Ventral Attention Network r	Association	Includes the temporo-parietal junction and ventral frontal cortex
Fronto-Parietal Network p	Association	Includes the dorsolateral prefrontal cortex, the inferior parietal lobule, and the middle temporal gyrus,
Limbic Network m	Association	Contains subcortical areas including amygdala, thalamus, basal ganglia, and cortical cingulate gyrus
Visual Network	Sensory-motor	Includes the striate and extrastriate cortical regions
Somato-Motor Network	Sensory-motor	Contains the primary motor and somato-sensory cortex

Table 1.
Major resting state networks of the human brain classified according to association or sensory-motor functions. Network identification follows that of Yeo et al., [53].

4. RSN dynamics and brain states

4.1 Assessing sources of connectivity modulation

While methodological advances in RS-fMRI have made significant strides in unveiling a macro-scale, network-based architecture for the brain, how brain functions emerge from network connectivity remains uncertain. Brain states like those of sleep or altered states of consciousness undergo continually changing dynamics involving whole brain networks. These dynamics are regularly modulated by internal fluctuations in activity that can affect sensory efferent or motor afferent activity [70, 71] and alter spatiotemporal patterning [72]. The ubiquity of these influences reveals that brain dynamics involve causal influences affecting network connectivity, which can be detected with BOLD fMRI [73]. Accordingly, recent developments in RS-fMRI seek to build on functional connectivity determinations by relating causal sources of connectivity changes to brain states and behavior. Network descriptions of these have been termed effective connectivity.

4.1.1 Effective connectivity

Effective connectivity presumes that efficient causes precede their effects and that these are revealed in the time domain. Because the functional coupling among neuronal populations changes as a function of processing demands [74] it is inherently context-dependent and dynamic. Accordingly, effective connectivity has been used to clarify sources of brain activity and the directionality of their influence. Inferences of causality are used to interpret the mechanisms that underlie neuronal dynamics and assist studies of how neuronal populations are functionally integrated [75]. In practice, models of effective connectivity seek to assess whether functional coupling is modulated under task-based manipulations and rely on fMRI data. The most common analytical methods include structural equation modeling (SEM), multivariate autoregressive models (MAR), GRANGER, and dynamic causal modeling (DCM).

DCM is perhaps the most widely employed approach for assessing effective connectivity and is based on an input-output model for a system of n interacting brain regions [76]. In this method, the activity of a neuronal population from each region is represented by a single state variable, which is perturbed by controlled inputs. DCM models report the series activity changes vis a vis the system's resting state represented by the system state vector (mathematical approximations of the system typically employ a Taylor series approximation that describes non-linear functions). Using these models it is possible to explore the dynamic character of brain activity under normal and pathological conditions. Unlike other approaches, DCM does not utilize time series data directly but combines a proposed model of the unknown neuronal dynamics with a forward model that translates neuronal states into output measurements. The description of the neuronal population activity employs a bilinear differential equation process, which is combined with the forward model.

Since the inception of the DCM, various methodological changes have extended the DCM approach [77, 78]. Recent, and more complex, models have included simulations from various prominent neuron classes, such as deep pyramidal cells, and spin stellate excitatory interneurons that contribute to the neuronal state [79]. Because of the complexity of these neuronal models, more general models have attempted to overcome their perceived difficulties in data fitting. One approach premises neural activity on generalized spiking described by Wilson Cowan spiking equations to satisfy a wider range of applications. In this adaptation, the Wilson Cowan equations are used to describe the evolution of excitatory and inhibitory activity in a population of neurons, instead of the bilinear equations used for both single and two- state DCM [80].

In a novel variant of DCM, effective connectivity analyses are conducted for large-scale or even whole-brain networks [81, 82]. This approach modifies the original DCM procedure in several ways: (i) translation of equations of state from the time to frequency domain using Fourier transformation, (ii) application of a mean field approximation across regions, and (iii) specification of conjugate priors on neuronal input. Choosing appropriate priors yield a generative model that can be used for making inferences about changes in directed connection strengths and inputs.

4.1.2 Granger causal analysis

Like DCM, Granger causal analysis provides a statistical tool for assessing directed functional connections from time series data, based on the concept that causes precede and induce their outcomes [13]. The method includes linear vector autoregressive models obtained from time series neural data, where a variable at a specific time point is modeled as a linearly weighted sum of its own past and that of a set of other variables, each represented by a vector. Minimizing estimation errors yields the set of optimal connection weights. Variable Y is said to be caused by variable X if the time series of X provides unique information not present in the prior Y series [83] that helps to predict the future Y series.

4.2 Macroscale brain organization and RSN dynamics

In principle, inferences of causality from directional connectivity determinations can be extended to brain-wide neuronal dynamics. Empirical studies from RS-fMRI, for example, show that RSNs are differentiated on the basis of their metastability and synchrony [84]. These and similar observations have stimulated models of brain function and behavior that predict that the human brain at rest operates at maximum metastability, that is, in a state of maximal network switching. Under such conditions, information flow can be said to be guided by temporally ordered sequences of metastable states [85, 86]. The existence of RSN properties like metastability thus implicates directed connectivity changes in the construction of brain states, which emerges from the dynamics of RSNs in whole brain, effective connectivity [87] in health, disease, or trauma. The methodological question that arises is that of generating a descriptive approach relating functional neuroimaging data to whole brain dynamics. Recent attempts to address this question have adopted two approaches.

4.2.1 Recurrence structure analysis

The first employs a BOLD, data-driven, computational method that leverages the method of *recurrence structure analysis* (RSA), a mathematical procedure derived from Poincare's recurrence theorem [15]. The Poincaré theorem states that trajectories of a complex dynamical system visit certain regions of their available state space more frequently over the course of time than other regions of the state space. This "recurrent" behavior can be described by a *recurrence plot method* (RP), which allows a matrix-based visualization of recurrent states. These latter are mapped into state space trajectories described by symbolic sequences [88]. Combining the structure-function modules of a brain hierarchical atlas with the optimized recurrent structures yields resting-state networks presumed to reflect time dependent, recurrent cognitive states.

4.2.2 Landscape of informational structures

The second approach posits the governance of RSN dynamics by a ground-state global attractor. This global ground state is mathematically described as a stable stationary solution representing a point of maximal stability in a landscape of stationary points (nodes) that information flows toward or away from [89]. Similar to whole-brain models, the description of this landscape consists of coupling local dynamics with anatomical brain connectivity. The stability and instability directions of each stationary point are characterized by non-stationary solutions entering or leaving these points, respectively. This provides a framework in which coupled systems of differential equations describe individual brain regions (nodes) in terms of other brain regions and with respect to the global ground state; hence, there exists a global structure linking all stationary points. Accordingly, such points can be ordered by their level of attraction or stability and characterized by various topological measures, for example, number of energy levels (NoEL) or sensitivity to perturbations (criticality) [90], based on connectivity data. This theoretical framework has been shown to successfully account for the highly structured dynamics arising from spontaneous brain activity in RSNs [91].

5. Resting state networks in disease

5.1 RS-fMRI studies in clinical diagnosis

Given the utility of RSNs for understanding the brain's functional organization in healthy individuals, RS-fMRI has also been exploited for determining how the brain's organization is modified as the result of trauma, degeneration, or disease [92]. A majority of RS-fMRI studies have consisted of comparisons of resting-state functional connectivity patterns between groups of normal subjects and those with neurological or psychiatric impairments [93], in part due to the relative ease with which these studies can be conducted. While changes in the correlation patterns of spontaneous activity have been reported in many cases, the consistency of the correlations has varied significantly with the disease type. Studies of the default mode network in AD, for example, generally yield consistent patterning whereas network patterns in other types of diseases, for example, schizophrenia, exhibit wide variation.

Underlying mechanisms and even diagnostic markers of these dysfunctions are in many cases unknown, moreover, a hindrance to assessing how functional network changes modify behavior. This obstacle could be partially surmounted by knowing how focal perturbations impact functional and task-based connectivity. Supporting this, neuroimaging studies show that localized changes in neural activity result in distinct activity and functional connectivity changes within and between networks [93, 94]. Mapping of whole-brain effects on RSNs due to local trauma may therefore reveal how RSNs are globally reorganized following these insults. For example, the characterization of large-scale deregulations in functional connectivity may emerge from studies of selective trauma in highly interconnected core regions [95].

5.2 RS-fMRI tools for stroke-induced changes in brain organization

With this as an objective, RS-fMRI technical and analytical procedures have been exploited to interrogate RSN-based changes that occur in stroke. By definition, stroke is a clinical syndrome characterized as an acute, focal neurological deficit that is the result of vascular injury (e.g., infarction, hemorrhage) within the central nervous system [96]. It is itself a major cause of death and disability across the globe. In adults worldwide, stroke is the chief cause of acquired physical disability, and the second leading cause of mortality in middle-to high-income countries. Because the disruption is usually sudden, stroke's effects on neural networks can be directly attributed to the focal impairment, rather than to more widely extended and long-term processes, such as degeneration. Stroke frequently results from ischemia, for instance, which deprives the supply of blood to adjacent cerebral tissue [17].

Assessing the spatial locus of a stroke-based lesion requires knowledge of the brain vasculature, which assists in co-localizing fiber pathways and structural connectivity. Anterior circulation, for example, includes regions supplied by the anterior and middle cerebral arteries, which contain the ophthalmic artery. Strokes occurring within the opthalmic artery lead to monocular loss of vision. Proximal occlusion of the middle cerebral artery, on the other hand, can cause contralateral hemiparesis and hemi-sensory loss, visual field defect, and/or hemineglect [96].

5.3 Connectivity determinations in stroke diagnosis

As mentioned, stroke outcomes involve not only focal disturbances at affected sites, that is, the set of regions directly damaged or indirectly affected by the stroke, but also those more distally located that are embedded within the larger functional network that is in dynamic balance with other networks of the brain. Hence, resting-state measures of connectivity can be expected to reflect a more distributed network organization than the lesion site alone and to be correspondingly seen in spatially extended, connectivity changes.

Consistent with this, global studies of focal infarcts affecting motor behaviors characteristically display a decrease in functional connectivity involving interhemispheric homologous sensory and motor areas, which is correlated with the degree of behavioral impairment. Reduced functional connectivity between hemispheres is also seen in rodent models of stroke [97], corresponding with decreases in motor proficiency [98]. In the first few days after stroke, this involves the connectivity between the ipsilesional primary sensorimotor cortex and its contralateral homologs [99]. Similarly, RS-fMRI of the sensorimotor network in humans, including the M1, SMA, secondary somatosensory cortex, cerebellum, putamen, and thalamus regions, reveals a direct correlation between motor performance and the degree of M1 interhemispheric connectivity [100]. Structural observations are consistent with this and show that the integrity of corticospinal fibers correlates with the reduction in interhemispheric M1 resting-state connectivity [99, 101]; RSN studies of effective connectivity with DCM further show that post-stroke excitatory, ipsilesional influences from premotor areas to M1 are also reduced, decreasing M1 output for paretic hand movements [17]. Ipsilesional inhibitory influences from M1 to the contralesional M1 are also attenuated. Together, these results implicate a reduction in inhibitory interhemispheric control of M1 homologs in paretic motor movements and excitatory intrahemispheric effects from premotor areas to M1. Importantly, they also reveal the interpretive utility of combining RS-fMRI effective and functional connectivity determinations in network assessments.

5.4 Assessing topological changes in stroke

Functional determinations assist in the identification of resting networks based on characterization of connectivity number, direction, and weight. Changes in such parameters help to assess the degree to which the network has retained its functional association; that is, the degree to which it is intact. On the other hand, they do not assess connectivity topography, which reflects how the organization of the network influences information flow, which needs to be assessed with graph theoretical parameters like centrality or modularity. Recent evidence in animal models notably indicates that network topology is likely to change following stroke [98]. In a mice model, total functional connectivity increases in comparison with normal controls. Since interhemispheric connectivity is reduced in most stroke subtypes, this suggests that intrahemispheric functional connectivity is cumulatively increased, generating a new organizational network structure within the affected hemisphere; that is, a transference of interhemispheric callosal connections to intrahemispheric targets.

Diagnostic assessments of network reorganization in stroke patients, accordingly, have been required, typically employing graph theoretic modular analysis. Modular analysis of task-based studies in normal subjects, for example, shows a high level of reorganization of nodes in the frontal and temporal cortices from the resting state.

Moreover, as mentioned, complex dynamics occur between networks during task performance, which involves the reallocation of network modules. Graph theoretic analysis shows that this entails the switching of network topologies between the frontoparietal, ventral attention, and the dorsal attention areas [63–65]. In like manner, modularity determinations can be expected to show stroke-induced reorganization.

Existing studies reveal, in fact, a low-dimensional architecture following stroke [57]. The significance of this network reorganization is as yet undetermined. One possibility is that decreased modularity reflects a default strategy for efficient behavioral responses in a complex environment, which is needed to reduce the degrees of freedom in movement [101]. In healthy individuals, a higher modularity provides for exploration of varied trajectories, that is, there is a maximizing of degrees of freedom, which needs to be reduced to provide stability for tasking. In stroke, this exploratory ability is lost, together with a corresponding loss in modularity. The reduction in modularity would thus imply a reduced ability to process information effectively [57].

Methodologically, assessing this possibility would require RS-fMRI procedures capable of whole-brain modeling to determine whether and which topographical adjustments occur on a global scale [90]. This is likely to require a synergy of ongoing developments that merge enhanced signal recognition and data acquisition, big data processing pipelines, and whole brain reconstruction [22, 50, 90], suggesting that advanced clinical analysis with RS-fMRI remains at an early, but promising stage.

6. Conclusion

Resting-state fMRI has enabled the identification of brain networks critical to affecting how humans interact, perceive, and process environmental and internal stimuli. Much of the success of this discovery can be attributed to the synergy between the technical capabilities of fMRI and the low-frequency activity characterizing RSNs. RS-fMRI has benefitted from a spectrum of technical advances in fMRI that have occurred since the initial discovery of RSNs, including improved data-gathering capacity, processing, and handling. The enhanced reliability of RSN detection made possible by these advances has underwritten increasingly powerful interpretive tools that are clarifying the role and structure of brain networks in organizing and executing global brain function. These insights into global brain events have in turn revealed areas where new technical advances, like big data processing and whole brain modeling, are needed, which can interrogate not only resting-state connectivity associations but also the dynamic variations in these associations that occur during brain behavior. While the use of these tools is currently limited to the research laboratory, their future potential for clinical use warrants the current expansion in technical development that will make possible the diagnosis of brain states.

DOI: http://dx.doi.org/10.5772/intechopen.113802

Author details

Denis Larrivee[1,2]

1 Mind and Brain Institute, University of Navarra Medical School, Spain

2 Loyola University Chicago, USA

*Address all correspondence to: sallar1@aol.com

References

[1] Biswal B, Yetkin FZ, Haughton VM, Hyde JS. Functional connectivity in the motor cortex of resting human brain using echo-planar MRI. Magnetic Resonance Medicine. 1995;**34**(4):537-541. DOI: 10.1002/mrm.1910340409

[2] van den Heuvel MP, Hilleke E, Hulshoff P. Exploring the brain network: A review on resting-state fMRI functional connectivity. European Neuropsychopharmacology. 2010;**20**:519-534

[3] Damoiseaux SA, Rombouts RB, Barkhof F, Beckman CF. Consistent resting-state networks across healthy subjects. National Academy of Sciences of the United States of America. 2006;**103**(37):13848-13853. DOI: 10.1073

[4] Seitzman BA, Snyder AZ, Leuthardt EC, Shimony JS. The state of resting state networks. Topics in Magnetic Resonance Imaging. 2019;**28**(4):189-196. DOI: 10.1097/RMR.0000000000000214

[5] Smitha KA, Akhil RK, Arun KM, et al. Resting state fMRI: A review on methods in resting state connectivity analysis and resting state networks. Neuroradiology Journal. 2017;**30**(4):305-317. DOI: 10.1177/1971400917697342

[6] Ogawa S, Tank DW, Menon R, et al. Intrinsic signal changes accompanying sensory stimulation: Functional brain mapping with magnetic resonance imaging. Proceedings of the National Academy of Science USA. 1992;**89**:5951-5955

[7] Bandettini P. The spatial, temporal, and interpretive limits of functional MRI. In: Davis K, Charney D, Coyle JT, Nemeroff C, editors. Neuropsychopharmacology: The Fifth Generation of Progress. Philadelphia: Lippincott, Williams, and Wilkins; 2002

[8] Kazan SM, Weiskopf N. fMRI Methods. Encyclopedia of Spectroscopy and Spectrometry (Third Edition). 2017:670-677. DOI: 10.1016/B978-0-12-409547-2.12109-2

[9] Loued-Khenissi L, Doll O, Preuschoff K. An overview of functional magnetic resonance imaging techniques for organizational research. Organizational Research Methods. 2019;**22**(1):17-45

[10] Biswal B. Resting state fMRI: A personal history. NeuroImage. 2012;**62**(2):938-944

[11] Deshmane ME, Gulani V, Griswold MA, Seiberlich N. Parallel MR imaging. Journal of Magnetic Resonance Imaging. 2012;**36**(1):55-72. DOI: 10.1002/jmri.23639

[12] Vadmal V, Junno G, Badye C, et al. MRI image analysis methods and applications. Neuro-Oncology Advances. 2020;**2**(1):1-13

[13] Seth AK, Barrett AB, Barnett L. Granger causality analysis in neuroscience and neuroimaging. The Journal of Neuroscience. 2015;**35**(8):3293-3297

[14] Friston KJ, Harrison L, Penny W. Dynamic causal modelling. NeuroImage. 2003;**19**:1273-1302

[15] Beim Graben P, Jimenez-Marin A, Diez I, Cortes JM, et al. Metastable resting state brain dynamics. Frontiers in Computational Neuroscience. 2019;**13**:62. DOI: 10.3389/fncom.2019.00062

[16] Fox MD, Greicius M. Clinical applications of resting state functional connectivity. Frontiers in Systems Neuroscience. 2010;**4**(19):1

[17] Rehme AK, Grefkes C. Cerebral network disorders after stroke: Evidence from imaging-based connectivity analyses of active and resting brain states in humans. Journal of Physiology. 2013;**591**(1):17-31

[18] Siegel JS, Ramsey LE, Snyder AZ, et al. Disruptions of network connectivity predict impairment in multiple behavioral domains after stroke. Proceedings of the National Academy of Sciences. 2016:E4367-E4376. DOI: 10.1073/pnas.1521083113

[19] Voss MW, Soto C, Yoo S, et al. Exercise and hippocampal memory systems. Trends in Cognitive Science. 2019;**23**(4):318-333. DOI: 10.1016/j.tics.2019.01.006

[20] Vizioli L, Moeller S, Dowdle L, et al. Lowering the thermal noise barrier in functional brain mapping with magnetic resonance imaging. Nature Communications. 2021;**12**:5181. DOI: 10.1038/s41467-021-25431-8

[21] Smith SM, Vidaurre D, Beckmann CF, et al. Functional connectomics from resting-state fMRI. Trends in Cognitive Science. 2013;**2013**(17):666-682. DOI: 10.1016/j.tics.2013.09.016

[22] Raimondo L, Ĺcaro AF, Jurjen HO, et al. Advances in resting state fMRI acquisitions for functional connectomics. NeuroImage. 2021;**243**:118503

[23] Yacoub E, Van De Moortele PF, Shmuel A, et al. Signal and noise characteristics of Hahn SE and GE BOLD fMRI at 7 T in humans. NeuroImage. 2005;**2005**(24):738-750. DOI: 10.1016/j.neuroimage

[24] Van Dijk KRA, Hedden T, Venkataraman A, et al. Intrinsic functional connectivity as a tool for human connectomics: Theory, properties, and optimization. Journal of Neurophysiology. 2010;**103**:297-321. DOI: 10.1152/jn.00783.2009

[25] Maknojia S, Churchill NW, Schweizer TA, Graham SJ. Resting state fMRI: Going through the motions. Frontiers in Neuroscience. 2019;**13**:825. DOI: 10.3389/fnins.2019.00825

[26] Yan CG, Craddock RC, Zuo XN, et al. Standardizing the intrinsic brain: Towards robust measurement of inter-individual variation in 1000 functional connectomes. NeuroImage. 2013;**80**:246-262

[27] Demetriou L, Kowalczyk OS, Tyson G, et al. A comprehensive evaluation of increasing temporal resolution with multiband- accelerated protocols and effects on statistical outcome measures in fMRI. NeuroImage. 2018;**176**:404-416. DOI: 10.1016/j.neuroimage.2018.05.011

[28] Preti MG, Bolton TA, Ville DV. The dynamic functional connectome: State-of- the-art and perspectives. NeuroImage. 2016:41-54. DOI: 10.1016/j.neuroimage.2016.12.061

[29] Zalesky A, Fornito A, Cocchi L, et al. Time-resolved resting-state brain networks. Proceedings of the National Academy of Science USA. 2014;**2014**(111):10341-10346. DOI: 10.1073/pnas.1400181111

[30] Aedo-Jury F, Schwalm M, Hamzehpour L, Stroh A. Brain states govern the spatio-temporal dynamics of resting-state functional connectivity. eLife. 2020;**22**(9):e53186. DOI: 10.7554/eLife.53186

[31] Jacobs HI, Priovoulos N, Poser BA, et al. Dynamic behavior of the locus coeruleus during arousal-related memory pro- cessing in a multi-modal 7T fMRI paradigm. eLife. 2020;**9**. DOI: 10.7554/eLife.52059

[32] Wu GR, Marinazzo D. Sensitivity of the resting-state haemodynamic response function estimation to autonomic nervous system fluctuations. Philosophical Transactions A. Mathematics, Physics and Engineering Science. 2016;**374**. DOI: 10.1098/rsta.2015.0190

[33] Chen JE, Polimeni JR, Bollmann S, Glover GH. On the analysis of rapidly sampled fMRI data. NeuroImage. 2019;**188**:807-820. DOI: 10.1016/j.neuroimage.2019.02.008

[34] Huotari N, Raitamaa L, Helakari H, et al. Sampling rate effects on resting state fMRI metrics. Frontiers in Neuroscience. 2019;**13**:279. DOI: 10.3389/fnins.2019.00279

[35] Barth M, Breuer F, Koopmans PJ, et al. Simultaneous multislice (SMS) imaging techniques. Magnetic Resonance Medicine. 2016;**2016**(75):63-81. DOI: 10.1002/mrm.25897

[36] Breuer FA, Blaimer M, Heidemann RM, et al. Controlled aliasing in parallel imaging results in higher accelera- tion (CAIPIRINHA) for multi-slice imaging. Magnetic Resonance Medicine. 2005;**53**:684-691. DOI: 10.1002/mrm.20401

[37] Setsompop K, Gagoski BA, Polimeni JR, et al. Blipped-controlled aliasing in parallel imaging for simultaneous multislice echo pla- nar imaging with reduced g-factor penalty. Magnetic Resonance in Medicine. 2012;**67**:1210-1224. DOI: 10.1002/mrm.23097

[38] Hamilton J, Franson D, Seiberlich N. Recent advances in parallel imaging for MRI. Progress in Nuclear Magnetic Resonance Spectroscopy. 2017;**101**:71-95. DOI: 10.1016/j.pnmrs.2017.04.002

[39] Calogero C. Recent advances in parallel imaging for MRI: WAVE-CAIPI technique. Journal of advanced. Health Care. 2022;**4**(1)

[40] Batson MA, Petridou N, Klomp DW, et al. Single session imaging of cerebellum at 7 tesla: Obtaining structure and function of multiple motor subsystems in individual subjects. PLoS One. 2015;**10**:e0134933. DOI: 10.1371/jour- nal.pone.0134933

[41] Zahneisen B, Hugger T, Lee KJ, et al. Single shot concentric shells trajectories for ultra fast fMRI. Magnetic Resonance Medicine. 2012;**68**:484-494. DOI: 10.1002/mrm.23256

[42] Akin B, Lee HL, Hennig J, et al. Enhanced subject-specific resting-state network detection and extraction with fast fMRI. Human Brain Mapping. 2017;**2017**(38):817-830. DOI: 10.1002/hbm.23420

[43] Pohmann R, Speck O, Scheffler K. 2016. Signal-to-noise ratio and MR tissue parameters in human brain imaging at 3, 7, and 9.4 tesla using current receive coil arrays. Magnetic Resonance Medicine. 2016;**75**:801-809. DOI: 10.1002/mrm.25677

[44] Vaughan JT, Garwood M, Collins CM, et al. 7T vs. 4T: RF power, homogeneity, and signal-to-noise comparison in head images. Magnetic Resonance Medicine. 2001;**46**:24-30. DOI: 10.1002/mrm.1156

[45] Branco P, Seixas D, Castro SL. Temporal reliability of ultra-high field resting- state MRI for single-subject

sensorimotor and language mapping. NeuroImage. 2018;**168**:499-508. DOI: 10.1016/j.neuroimage.2016.11.029

[46] Torrisi S, Nord CL, Balderston NL, et al. Resting state connectivity of the human habenula at ultra-high field. NeuroImage. 2017;**147**:872-879. DOI: 10.1016/j.neuroimage.2016.10.034

[47] Van de Moortele PF, Auerbach EJ, Olman C, et al. T1 weighted brain images at 7 tesla unbiased for proton density, T2* contrast and RF coil receive B1 sensitivity with simultaneous vessel visualization. NeuroImage. 2009;**46**:432-446. DOI: 10.1016/j.neuroimage.2009.02.009

[48] Van Essen DC, Ugurbil K, Auerbach E, et al. The human connectome project: A data acquisition perspective. NeuroImage. 2012;**62**(4):2222-2231

[49] Biswal BB, Mennes M, Zuo XN, et al. Toward discovery science of human brain function. National Academy of Sciences of the United States of America. 2010;**107**(10):4734-4739

[50] Phinyomark A, Ibanez-Marcelo E, Petri G. Resting-state fMRI functional connectivity: Big data preprocessing pipelinesand topological data analysis. IEEE Transactions on Big Data. 2017;**3**(4):415-428

[51] Churchill NW et al. Optimizing preprocessing and analysis pipelines for single-subject fMRI. I. Standard temporal motion and physiological noise correction methods. Human Brain Mapping. 2012;**33**(3):609-627

[52] Ghrist B. Barcodes: The persistent topology of data. Bulletin of the American Mathematics Society. 2008;**45**(1):61-75

[53] Yeo BTT, Krienen FM, Sepulcre J, et al. The organization of the human cerebral cortex estimated by intrinsic functional connectivity. Journal of Neurophysiology. 2011;**106**:1125-1165. DOI: 10.1152/jn.00338.2011

[54] Shahhosseini Y, Miranda MF. Functional connectivity methods and their applications in fMRI data. Entropy. 2022;**24**:390. DOI: 10.3390/e24030390

[55] Le Q, Karpenko A, Ngiam J, and Ng A. ICA with reconstruction cost for efficient overcomplete feature learning. In: Shawe-Taylor J, Zemel R, Bartlett P, Pereira F, Weinberger KQ, editors, Advances in Neural Information Processing Systems. Vol. 4. New York: Curran Associates, Inc.; 2011

[56] Yang J, Gohel S, Vachha B. Current methods and new directions in resting state fMRI. Clinical Imaging. 2020;**65**:47-53. DOI: 10.1016/j.clinimag.2020.04.004

[57] Corbetta M, Siegel JS, Schulman GL. On the low dimensionality of behavioral deficits and alterations of brain network connectivity after focal injury. Cortex. 2018;**107**:229-237

[58] Crossley NA, Mechelli A, Vertes PE, et al. Cognitive relevance of the community structure of the human brain functional coactivation network. Proceedings of the National Academy of Sciences USA. 2013;**110**:11583-11588

[59] Lerman-Sinkoff DB, Barch DM. Network community structure alterations in adult schizophrenia: Identification and localization of alterations. Neuroimage Clinic. 2016;**10**:96-106. DOI: 10.1016/j.nicl.2015.11.011

[60] Bordier C, Nicolini C, Forcellini G, Bifone A. Disrupted modular organization of primary sensory brain areas in schizophrenia. Neuroimage

Clinic. 2018;**18**:682-693. DOI: 10.1016/j.nicl.2018.02.035

[61] Bullmore ET, Sporns O. Complex brain networks: Graph theoretical analysis of structural and functional systems. Nature Review Neuroscience. 2009;**10**:186-198. DOI: 10.1038/nrn2575

[62] Liang X, Zou QH, He Y, Yang YH. Topologically reorganized connectivity architecture of default-mode, executive-control, and salience networks across working memory task loads. Cerebral Cortex. 2016;**26**:1501-1511. DOI: 10.1093/cercor/bhu316

[63] Fornito A, Harrison BJ, Zalesk A, Simons JS. Competitive and cooperative dynamics of large-scale brain functional networks supporting recollection. National Academy of Sciences of the United States of America. 2012;**109**(31):12788-12793

[64] Bray S, Arnold AEGF, Levy RM, Iaria G. Spatial and temporal functional connectivity changes between resting and attentive states. Human Brain Mapping. 2015;**36**:549-565. DOI: 10.1002/hbm.22646

[65] Vatansever D, Menon DK, Manktelow AE, et al. Default mode network connectivity during task execution. NeuroImage. 2015;**2015**(122):96-104. DOI: 10.1016/j.neuroimage.2015.07.053

[66] Braun U, Schafer A, Walter H, et al. Dynamic reconfiguration of frontal brain networks during executive cognition in humans. Proceedings of the National Academy of Science USA. 2015;**112**:11678-11683. DOI: 10.1073/pnas.1422487112

[67] Leech R, Kamourieh S, Beckmann CF, Sharp DJ. Fractionating the default mode network: Distinct contributions of the ventral and dorsal posterior cingulate cortex to cognitive control. Journal of Neuroscience. 2011;**31**:3217-3224. DOI: 10.1523/jneurosci.5626-10.2011

[68] Rubinov M, Sporns O. Weight-conserving characterization of complex functional brain networks. NeuroImage. 2011;**56**:2068-2079. DOI: 10.1016/j.neuroimage.2011.03.069

[69] Lebedev AV, Nilsson J, Lövdén M. Working memory and reasoning benefit from different modes of large-scale brain dynamics in healthy older adults. Journal of Cognitive Neuroscience. 2018;**30**:1033-1046. DOI: 10.1162/jocn_a_01260

[70] Pachitariu M, Lyamzin DR, Lesica SM. State dependent population coding in primary auditory cortex. Journal of Neuroscience. 2015;**35**:2058-2073. DOI: 10.1523/jneurosci.3318-14.2015

[71] Schwalm M, Schmid F, Wachsmud L, et al. Cortext wide BOLD fMRI acti vity reflects locally recorded slow oscillation associated calcium waves. eLife. 2017;**6**:e27602

[72] Pais-Roldan P, Takahashi K, Sobczak F, et al. Indexing brain state dependent pupil dynamics with simultaneous fMRI and optical fiber calcium recording. National Academy of Sciences of the United States of America. 2020;**117**:6875-6882

[73] Staresina BP, Alink A, Kriegeskorte N, Henson RN. Awake reactivation predicts memory in humans. National Academy of Sciences of the United States of America. 2013;**110**:21159-21164

[74] Stephan KE, Friston KJ. Analyzing effective connectivity with functional magnetic resonance imaging.

Wiley Interdisciplinary Review of Cognitive Science. 2010;**1**(3):446-459. DOI: 10.1002/wcs.58

[75] Friston KJ. Functional and effective connectivity: A review. Brain Connectomics. 2011;**1**(1):13-36. DOI: 10.1089/brain.2011.0008

[76] Kiebel SJ, Garrido MI, Moran RJ, et al. Dynamic causal modelling for EEG and MEG. Cognitive Neurodynamics. 2008;**2**:121-136. DOI: 10.1007/s11571-008-9038-0

[77] Moran R, Pinotsis DA, Friston K. Neural masses and fields in dynamic causal modeling. Frontiers in Computational Neuroscience. 2013;**7**(57):1-12. DOI: 10.3389/fncom.2013.00057

[78] Wei H, Jafarian A, Zeidman P, et al. Bayesian fusion and multimodal DCM for EEG and fMRI. NeuroImage. 2020;**211**:6595

[79] Hass J, Hertäg L, Durstewitz D. A detailed data-driven network model of prefrontal cortex reproduces key features of in vivo activity. PLoS Computational Biology. 2016;**12**:e1004930. DOI: 10.1371/journal.pcbi.1004930

[80] Frässle S, Lomakina EI, Kasper L, et al. A generative model of whole-brain effective connectivity. NeuroImage. 2018;**179**:505-529. DOI: 10.1016/j.neuroimage.2018.05.058

[81] Frässle S, Lomakina EI, Razi A, et al. Regression DCM for fMRI. NeuroImage. 2017;**155**:406-421. DOI: 10.1016/j.neuroimage.2017.02.090

[82] Barnett L, Barrett AB, Seth AK. Granger causality and transfer entropy are equivalent for gaussian variables. Physics Review Letters. 2009;**103**:238701

[83] Lee WH, Frangou S. Linking functional connectivity and dynamic properties of resting-state networks. Scientific Reports. 2017;**7**:16610. DOI: 10.1038/s41598-017-16789-1

[84] Rabinovich MI, Huerta R, Varona P, Afraimovich VS. Transient cognitive dynamics, metastability, and decision making. PLoS Computational Biology. 2008;**4**(5):e1000072. DOI: 10.1371/journal.pcbi.1000072

[85] Tognoli E, Kelso JA. The metastable brain. Neuron. 2014;**81**(1):35-48. DOI: 10.1016/j.neuron.2013.12.022

[86] Tagliazucchi E, Laufs H. Decoding wakefulness levels from typical fMRI resting-state data reveals reliable drifts between wakefulness and sleep. Neuron. 2014;**82**(3):695-708. DOI: 10.1016/j.neuron.2014.03.020

[87] Beim Graben P, Sellers KK, Fröhlich F, Hutt A. Optimal estimation of recurrence structures from time series. Europhysics Letters. 2016;**2016**(114):38003. DOI: 10.1209/0295-5075/114/38003

[88] Carvalho A, Langa J, Robinson J. Attractors for infinite-dimensional non-autonomous dynamical systems. In: Applied Mathematical Sciences. New York: Springer; 2012

[89] Soler-Toscano F, Galad'ı JA, Escrichs A, et al. What lies underneath: Precise classification of brain states using time-dependent topological structure of dynamics. PLoS Computational Biology. 2022;**18**(9):e1010412. DOI: 10.1371/journal.pcbi.1010412

[90] López-González A, Panda R, Ponce-Alvarez A, et al. Loss of consciousness reduces the stability of brain hubs and the heterogeneity of brain dynamics. Communications Biology. 2021;**4**(1):1037-1052

[91] Greicius M. Resting-state functional connectivity in neuropsychiatric disorders. Current Opinion in Neurology. 2008;**21**:424-430

[92] Andoh J, Matsushita R, Zatorre RJ. Asymmetric interhemispheric transfer in the auditory network: Evidence from tms, resting-state fMRI, and diffusion imaging. Journal of Neuroscience. 2015;**35**(43):14602-14611. DOI: 10.1523/jneurosci.2333-15.2015

[93] Watanabe T, Hirose S, Wada H, et al. A pairwise maximum entropy model accurately describes resting-state human brain networks. Nature Communications. 2013;**4**:1370

[94] Aerts H, Fias W, Caeyenberghs K, et al. Brain networks under attack: Robustness properties and the impact of lesions. Brain. 2016;**139**(12):3063-3083. DOI: 10.1093/brain/aww194

[95] Murphy SJX, Werring DJ. Stroke: Causes and clinical features. Medicine. 2020;**48**:9561

[96] Rehme AK, Eickhoff SB, Rottschy C, et al. Activation likelihood estimation meta-analysis of motor-related neural activity after stroke. NeuroImage. 2012;**59**:2771-2782

[97] Hall GR, Kaiser M, Farr TD. Functional connectivity change in response to stroke is comparable across species from mouse to man. Stroke. 2021;**52**:2961-2963

[98] van Meer MP, Otte WM, van der Marel K, et al. Extent of bilateral neuronal network reorganization and functional recovery in relation to stroke severity. The Journal of Neuroscience. 2012;**32**:4495-4507. DOI: 10.1523/jneurosci.3662-11.2012

[99] Carter AR, Astafiev SV, Lang CE, et al. Resting interhemispheric functional magnetic resonance imaging connectivity predicts performance after stroke. Annals of Neurology. 2010;**67**:365-375

[100] Carter AR, Patel KR, Astafiev SV, et al. Upstream dysfunction of somatomotor functional connectivity after corticospinal damage in stroke. Neurorehabilitation and Neural Repair. 2012;**26**:7-19

[101] Santello M. Getting a grasp of theories of sensorimotor control of the hand: Identification of underlying neural mechanisms. Motor Control. 2015;**19**(2):149-153. DOI: 10.1123/mc.2014-0057

Section 4

Multi-Parametric Tissue Specific MRI Procedures

Chapter 6

Advantages of Digital Technology in the Assessment of Bone Marrow Involvement by Magnetic Resonance Images

Pilar Giraldo Castellano and Mercedes Roca Espiau

Abstract

Magnetic resonance imaging (MRI) is the gold standard for evaluating bone marrow (BM). The information provided is a useful tool for obtaining a global map of the contents of the medullary cavity. The applications of this technique to the study of different processes affecting the bone marrow are of great importance to know the extension of disease, to distinguish by image different entities, and to evaluate response to therapies. Actually, machine learning tools aid in the interpretation of images and patterns that are not visible or are unfamiliar to the observer. In addition, integrating clinical, biological, and therapeutic data with imaging using artificial intelligence methods applied to these studies provides a broad perspective and tool that can predict the risk of complications. The systematic inclusion of structured bone marrow MRI reporting is useful to standardize the collected data collaborate in developed algorithms to learning model, and facilitate clinical management and academics collaboration.

Keywords: bone marrow, MRI, infiltration patterns, lysosomal disorders, structured reports, machine learning

1. Introduction

This chapter reviews the information provided by magnetic resonance imaging (MRI) as a useful tool to obtain a global map of the content of the medullary cavity and the applications of the technique to the study of different processes affecting bone marrow.

The daily clinical practice involves resolving situations of uncertainty in order to obtain the most accurate diagnosis possible and initiate therapeutic measures quickly. In this sense, the exchange of information and collaboration between the clinical physician and the MRI specialist is essential to answer questions regarding the global or focal involvement of the bone marrow in various pathological situations.

MRI, as a useful imaging technique to distinguish differences and anomalies in different tissues, bases its resolution on reflecting the balance between the medullary fatty component and the hematopoietic cellular component, providing an image of the variations that occur between these components within the bone cavity [1].

Artificial intelligence (AI) models based on deep learning algorithms offer actually diagnostic assessment and follow-up assistance for low-frequency entities, with findings to date suggesting that the diagnostic performance of such systems is equivalent to that of health-care professionals [2].

2. Rational basis of magnetic resonance imaging

The physical basis of the procedure is due to the property possessed by some atomic nuclei of orientation in a magnetic field and the emission of a signal when subjected to an electromagnetic wave of an appropriate frequency. The basis is sending a sound signal on a magnetized object, developing macroscopic magnetization phases, which disturb the state of equilibrium due to the sound signal and collection of the MR signal and the return to the state of equilibrium or relaxation. This signal of a return to equilibrium or relaxation is the MR signal [3].

Some notions to keep in mind are the following:

- The relaxation phenomenon characterizes the times T1 and T2.
- The repetition time or TR is the interval that separates 2 impulses/2 successive.
- The echo time or TE is the time interval separating the impulse/2 from the measurement of the emitted signal.
- The longitudinal relaxation time or T1 represents the growth of the magnetism M (Mz component) to return to its initial value. It is an exponential growth, which takes place slowly.
- The transverse relaxation time or T2 represents the decrease of the vector M (Mxy component) to return to its initial value. It occurs rapidly and is linked to the loss of proton coherence.
- T1-weighted sequences provide information on anatomical landmarks, and T2 sequences provide a closer approximation to the histological characterization of the involvement.
- The STIR sequence adds a fat suppression effect and chemical shift artifact elimination. It combines a short T1 with a long TR and shows a contrast between healthy and pathologic tissue superior to conventional T2.
- In phase-out-of-phase: Due to its lack of proton content, the trabecular bone does not present an MR signal but creates heterogeneities in the magnetic field. This is more evident in Gradient echo sequences where this artifact can be contributory. Therefore, if the trabeculae have been destroyed, the artifact is smaller, and the signal intensity will be higher.
- Diffusion-weighted MR imaging (DWI) is a technique that assesses motion of watermolecules in the soft tissues, known as Brownian motion, for tissue

characterization. A DWI sequence may be helpful for lesion detection, but its utility in evaluating and characterizing focal bone marrow lesions is unknown. MR Spectroscopy. MRS is useful for fat quantification, and bone marrow studies have primarily focused on its use in the imaging of osteoporosis [4].

3. Applications of magnetic resonance imaging to the study of bone marrow

In general, bone marrow involvement is easy to detect and interpret by MRI without requiring sophisticated sequences; it is very useful to obtain a map of hematopoietic marrow distribution and infiltration.

3.1 Normal bone marrow distribution

In children, bone marrow occupies 85% of the bone and accounts for 5% of the body weight. In the adult, red marrow is located in vertebrae, sternum, ribs, epiphyses of long bones, and iliac crests.

The bone marrow content in adults is 70% water and 30% fat. Hematopoietic marrow (red) consists of 40% water, 40% fat, and 20% protein. The fatty marrow (yellow) is made up of 15% water, 85% fat, and 5% protein.

Normal bone always contains both fat and red marrow, the percentage depending on age and anatomical region (**Figure 1**). However, it undergoes variations in its fatty composition/hematopoietic cellularity as part of a transformation phenomenon and in dependence on cellular requirements. Fat tissue is very labile and can be replaced by hematopoietic tissue under the influence of appropriate stimuli. Anatomically,

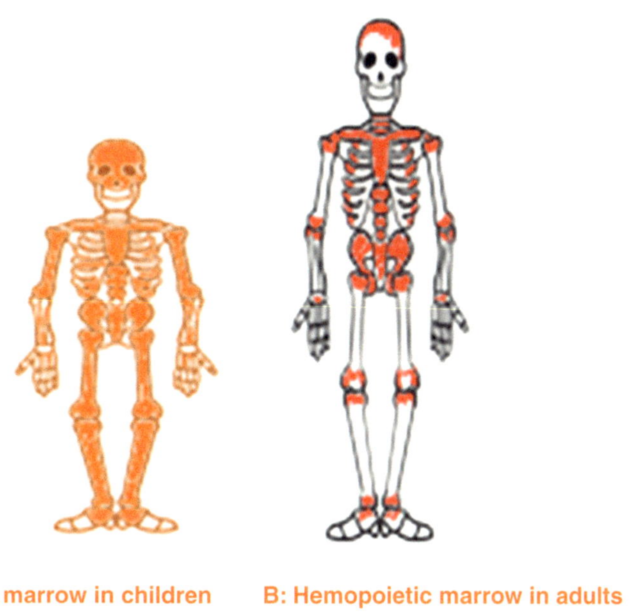

Figure 1.
Distribution of red marrow and fat. A in the child. Red bone marrow is distributed in 85% of the bones. B in the adult, the red bone marrow is located in vertebrae, sternum, ribs, epiphyses of long bones, and iliac crests.

medullary repopulation occurs in the reverse direction of regression, i.e., from proximal to distal areas.

MRI is able to reflect the ratio between the medullary fatty and hematopoietic components, through the changes that occur within the bone cavity [5, 6].

Marrow fat has a signal analogous to subcutaneous fat, the signal intensity is high due to its high proton content, expressing itself with a short T1 and a long T2 with high signal intensity in T1 and T2. As we have said, normal bone marrow contains 70% water and 30% fat and is hypointense in T1 and T2. T1 is the fundamental sequence for the study of bone marrow. The bone cortex has low proton content and small signal intensity.

Fat has a high signal in T1 and T2. Red marrow has an intermediate signal lower than fat and higher than muscle. The alterations that can occur are reconversion, infiltration, depletion, edema, and ischemia [7].

3.2 Patterns of bone marrow infiltration by MRI

The distribution of bone marrow involvement may be diffuse or focal. Several distribution patterns have been described according to the images that appear on magnetic resonance imaging. **Table 1** shows the patterns described by Moulopoulos et al. [8] in the study of the bone marrow in patients with bone marrow involvement and the one described by our group [9] (**Figure 2**).

3.3 Hematological entities with preferential involvement of bone marrow

3.3.1 Multiple myeloma (MM)

Eighty percent of patients with multiple myeloma present osteolytic lesions or demineralization at the time of diagnosis [10]. When these lesions become evident on radiography, more than 50% of the bone is already occupied.

There are three described patterns of infiltration in MM by MRI [11]:

1. Focal lesions, associated with lytic lesions in radiology, are the most frequent (**Figure 2**).

2. Diffuse infiltration appears in 25% of patients and is associated with decreased hemoglobin and a high percentage of medullary plasmacytosis. The MR signal is hypointense in T1 with diffuse gadolinium uptake (**Figure 3**).

According to Moulopoulos et al. [8]	According to Roca et al. [9]
Focal	Homogeneous (H)
Variegated (or variegata)	Nonhomogeneous (NH):
Diffuse	reticular (NHR)
	mottled (NHM)
	diffuse (NHD)

Table 1.
Patterns of bone marrow infiltration by MRI.

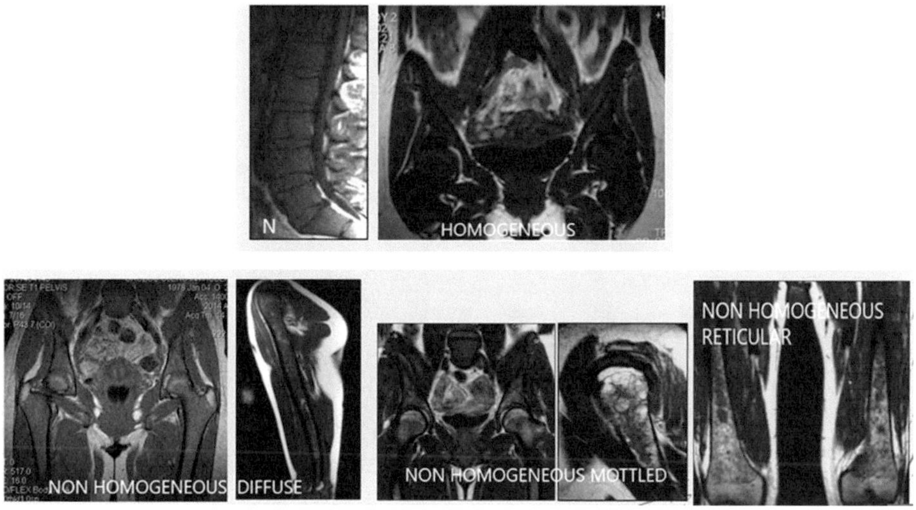

Figure 2.
Bone marrow infiltration. MRI patterns described by Roca-Espiau et al. 2007. Three MRI patterns were defined: Normal, homogeneous, and nonhomogeneous infiltration subtypes reticular, mottled, and diffuse.

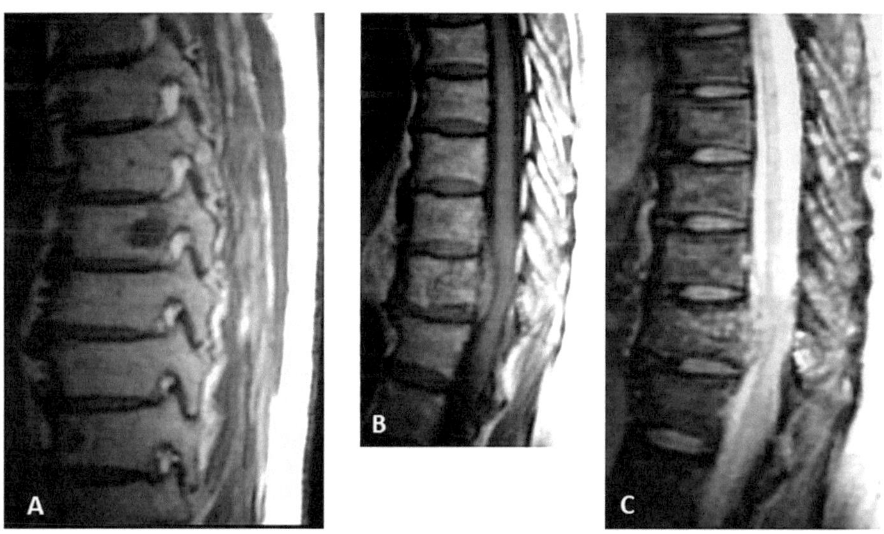

Figure 3.
Sagital spin echo (SE) T1 (A) focal pattern in spine in multiple myeloma. It is the most frequent lesions and corresponds to lytic images in plain radiology. SE T1 (B) and T2 (C) spine with diffuse infiltration. The MR signal is hypointense in T1.

3. Mottled or variegated pattern, with hypointense foci in T1 and generally hyperintense in T2 and STIR with contrast uptake (**Figure 4**). Libshitz et al. [12] describe diffuse involvement as areas where myeloma cells mix with hematopoietic cells, producing a displacement of hematopoiesis caused by nodular accumulations formed mainly by plasma cells. For this reason, the appearance of MRI is variable.

A strong association between diffuse infiltration and disease progression has been described. Diffuse infiltration is an unfavorable prognostic factor in patients with

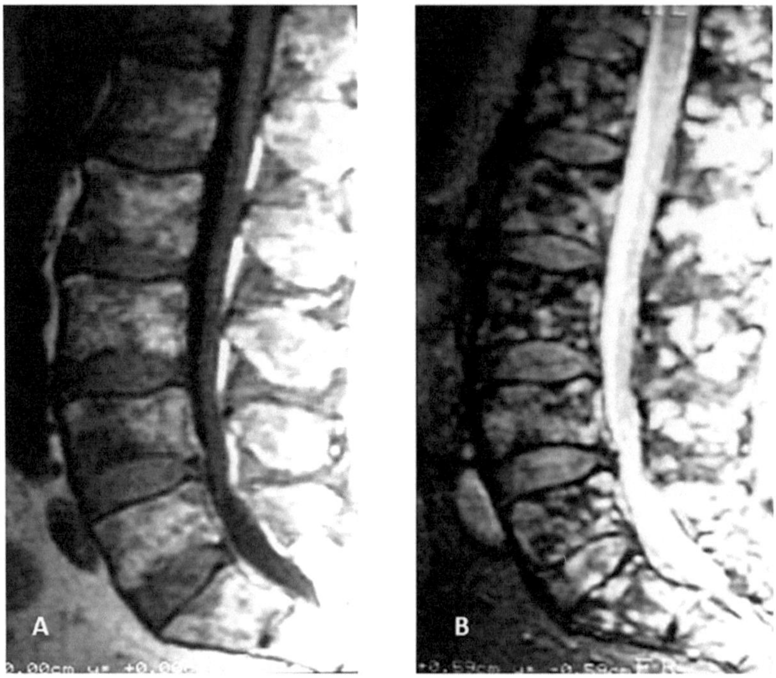

Figure 4.
Sagital spin echo (SE) T1 (A) and T2 (B) mottled or variegated pattern in multiple myeloma, with hypointense foci in T1 and hyperintense in T2.

normal bone radiology [13]. Approximately 15% of patients are asymptomatic at the time of diagnosis, but bone marrow infiltration can already be detected in up to 29–50% of patients [11–14]. Patients with focal and diffuse MR patterns tend to progress more rapidly than patients with mottled patterns. Following these criteria, MR infiltration imaging helps to identify patients who are at higher risk of complications and to predict disease progression [15, 16]. However, in the current diagnostic criteria for MM, only the focal pattern on MRI (> 1) is considered as a criterion for multiple myeloma (previously called symptomatic myeloma) and, therefore, an indication for treatment [16, 17].

MRI is probably not the most sensitive imaging procedure in the follow-up of the response in MM, since bone lesions will persist over time, and it is not possible to delimit whether it is an active lesion. It is, however, useful for comparative assessment of lesion progression [18, 19].

In the variety of light chain multiple myeloma, a different MRI pattern of mottled appearance with hypointense foci in both T1 and T2 have been described, analogous to the pattern that appears in Gaucher disease [20]. The diagnosis of solitary plasmacytoma requires histologic demonstration of plasma cell infiltration. Although radiotherapy can eradicate this lesion, most patients progress to multiple myeloma, which has been attributed to occult disease growth [21].

For this reason, MRI is important in the extension study, since it detects unsuspected lesions, especially at the vertebral level. Currently, the accepted treatment for these lesions is radiotherapy covering at least 2 cm outside the tumor, and for this purpose, it is recommended to perform a previous MRI of the plasmacytoma area.

The consensus panel (International Myeloma Workshop 2011) [22] recommends MRI in three situations:

- Asymptomatic myeloma (smoldering myeloma) to detect occult lesions.

- In symptomatic, for visualization of unsuspected focal lesions and soft tissue plasmacytomas in the spine and pelvis.

- In symptomatic, to predict evolution, according to the MRI pattern.

3.3.2 Non-Hodgkin's lymphoma and Hodgkin's lymphoma

Bone marrow infiltration occurs in 5–15% of patients with Hodgkin's lymphoma and in 25–40% of patients diagnosed with non-Hodgkin's lymphoma. In T1, the pattern of involvement is heterogeneous diffuse, with focal infiltration being less frequent. In T2, hypersignal is observed, as well as contrast uptake after gadolinium injection. This aspect is nonspecific and indistinguishable from other spinal cord infiltration of other origins, and there is no difference in the MRI pattern between the different histological types of lymphoma [23, 24] (**Figure 5**).

Due to the permeative nature of lymphomas, tumor extension can be observed in the form of a soft tissue mass without rupture of the bone cortex. Although it is not pathognomonic, since it can exist in other malignant lesions, especially in small cell tumors, its detection, and evaluation with MRI is highly suggestive of lymphoma [25].

3.3.3 Chronic myeloproliferative neoplasms

3.3.3.1 Polycythemia vera

In polycythemia rubra vera, the bone marrow of the axial skeleton appears hypointense in T1 with a diffuse and homogeneous character in MRI studies, being

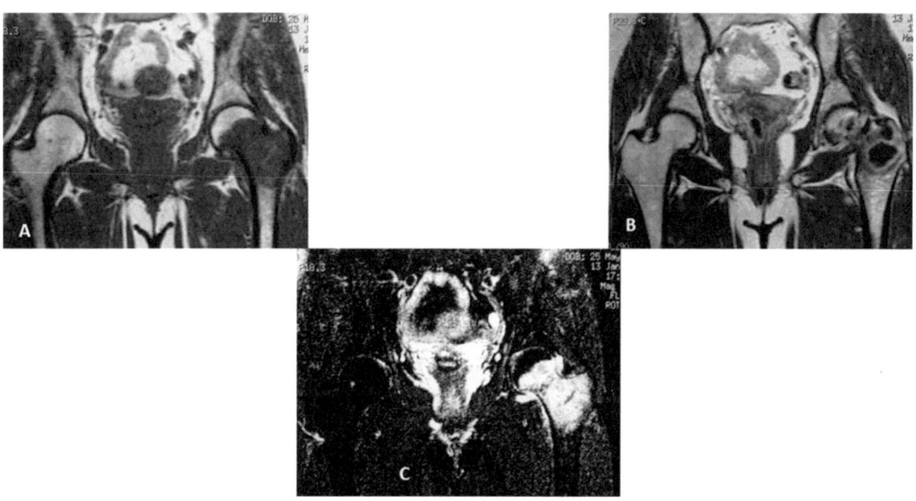

Figure 5.
Coronal pelvis spin echo (SE) T1 (A), T1 Gadolinio (B), and T2 FSat (C) in non-Hodgkin lymphoma. Pattern heterogeneous diffuse in T1, hyperintensity of signal in T2, contrast uptake after gadolinium injection.

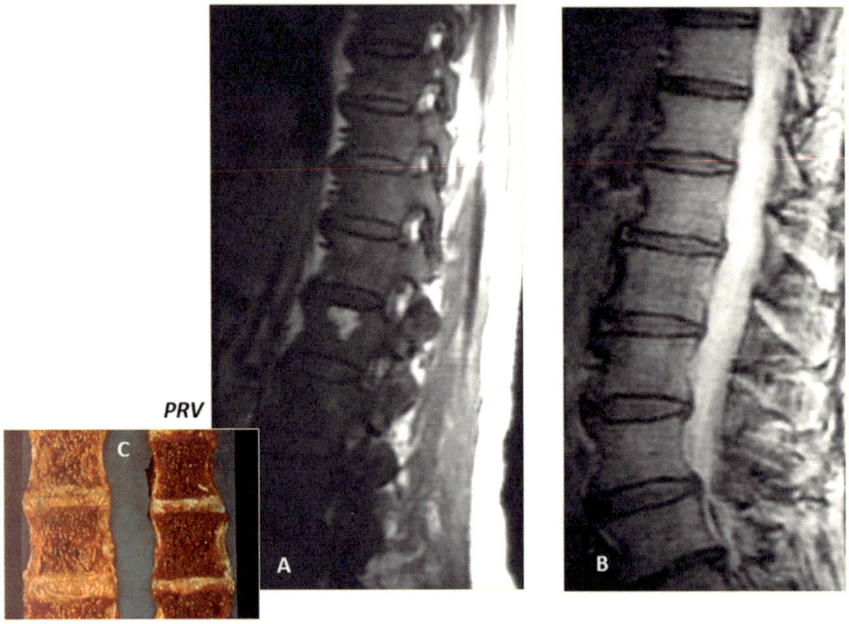

Figure 6.
Sagital spin echo (SE) T1 (A) and T2 (B) diffuse pattern in chronic myeloproliferative neoplasia (polycythemia rubra vera (PRV)). (C) Macroscopic section of spine with red infiltration PRV (right image) versus normal (left image).

indistinguishable from the diffuse involvement observed in other myeloproliferative neoplasia. When the reconversion is pronounced, the proximal epiphyses of the femur and humerus and the greater trochanter, also participate in the reconversion showing hyposignal in T1. In T2, the behavior can be variable depending on the cellularity, the extent of reticulin fibrosis, and the paramagnetic effect of iron if hemosiderosis is present (**Figure 6**). The assessment in the proximal femur can be quantified according to the involvement of the femoral head and greater trochanter. The greater trochanter is more resistant to reconversion than the epiphyses. Patients with infiltration of both have higher disease activity [26, 27].

3.3.3.2 Myelofibrosis

The fibrotic medulla, typical of primary or secondary myelofibrosis, is visualized in MRI as low signal areas in all sequences, but its appearance is nonspecific as in the rest of hematologic diseases and does not differentiate primary from secondary myelofibrosis. There is usually contrast uptake due to increased capillaries, large sinusoids, and increased vascular permeability [28]. Our group has performed a comparative study in patients diagnosed with primary or secondary myelofibrosis between histological findings and the pattern of bone marrow involvement by MRI. The results showed that the bone marrow patterns defined from lesser to a greater degree of involvement were: normal patterns according to age (NP), hematopoietic hyperplasia (HHP), reticular infiltration pattern (RP), mottled infiltration pattern (MP), diffuse heterogeneous infiltration pattern (DHI) and diffuse homogeneous infiltration pattern (HP) [29] (**Figure 7**).

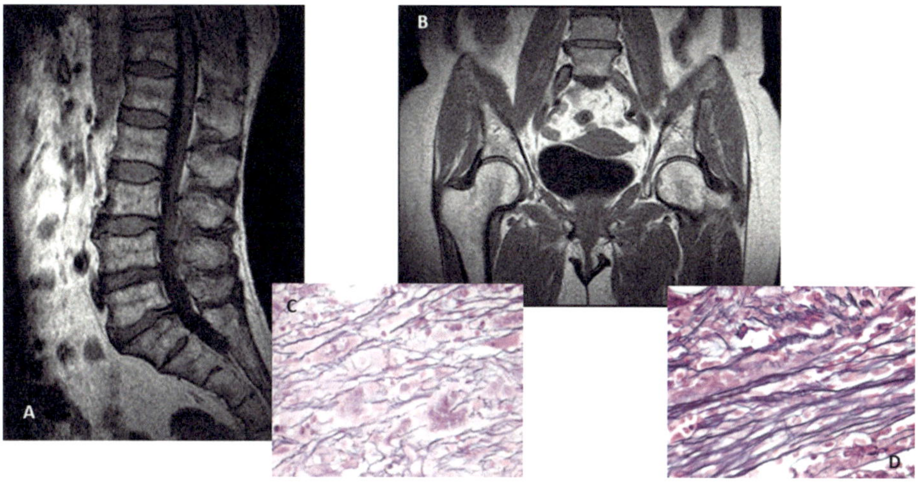

Figure 7.
Sagital spin echo (SE) T1 (A) mottled pattern, coronal SET1 (B) reticular pattern in chronic myeloproliferative neoplasia (myelofibrosis). (C) Bone marrow histological section (reticulin staining) showed reticular fibers. (D) Collagen fibers.

3.3.3.3 Systemic mastocytosis

Systemic mastocytosis is also a rare disease (less than 10% of mastocytosis), which usually affects adults and presents bone alterations in 70% of patients [26]. It has a special tropism for the axial skeleton, and although it can be silent, about 28% of patients report pain. The changes observed in simple radiology are small lytic or sclerotic lesions of focal or diffuse character (**Figure 8**). Mast cell proliferation in the

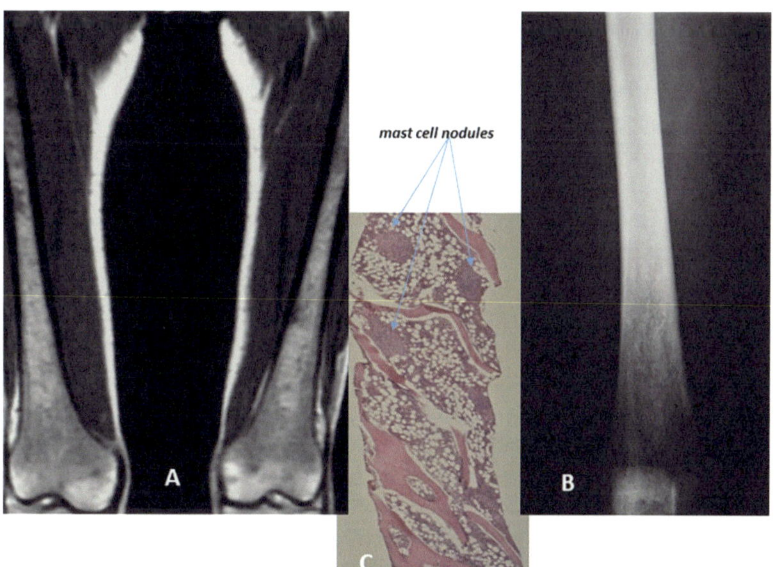

Figure 8.
Coronal spin echo (SE) T1 (A) fémurs heterogeneous reticular pattern in systemic mastocytosis. (B) Plain radiology of the femur (C). Bone marrow histological section (hematoxylin–eosin staining. HE×4). ↓ Showed mast cell nodules.

bone marrow stimulates fibroblastic activity with granulomatous reaction, resulting in trabecular destruction with replacement by neoformed bone. Soft tissue masses and deformities secondary to fractures may also be observed. MRI shows hypointense lesions in all sequences with diffuse distribution and homogeneous or mottled character that affect the axial skeleton and may extend to femurs and proximal humerus [30]. In any case, the infiltration presents a nonspecific signal, although sometimes it is not detectable by other diagnostic means [31].

3.3.4 Bone marrow aplasia and hypoplasia

Acquired aplasia is of unknown cause and may be secondary to chemical agents, drugs, or infectious agents. Some cases are irreversible. Biopsy is usually diagnostic, demonstrating the absence of cells or marked hypocellularity with the predominance of fatty marrow and fibrosis [32]. It should be kept in mind that areas of increased hematopoiesis may coexist with hypo- or acellular marrow, so that bone marrow biopsy from the iliac crest is a sample that does not always reflect the true state of marrow function. The marrow findings in cases of aplasia secondary to chemotherapy or irradiation may be diffuse or focal in cases of selective irradiation [33].

Hypocellular or aplastic marrow is characterized by a diffuse or mottled hyperintense pattern in T1, which corresponds to cellular replacement by fatty marrow. This signal enhancement is more appreciable in areas that normally contain red marrow remnants such as the proximal femur or vertebrae. In the appendicular skeleton, it is more difficult to appreciate this variation.

When there is a response to treatment, a heterogeneous pattern is observed in the vertebral bodies formed by hypointense foci in T1 and T2 that represent foci of hematopoiesis. MRI is a good method for assessing response to treatment [34, 35], taking into account that sometimes, these foci appear in vertebrae and are not seen in the pelvis, where the biopsy is normally performed if the patient recovers completely from his aplasia, the marrow returns to the normal appearance and distribution for his age.

The administration of erythropoiesis-stimulating factors as an adjuvant to chemotherapy treatment produces a patchy pattern in MRI showing hypointense foci in T1, which in T2 present identical or slightly increased signal, similar to hematopoietic foci in their behavior but located in areas where fatty marrow is normally present.

The depletion of medullary cellularity also occurs during ionizing irradiation at therapeutic doses. In vertebral irradiation, no signal changes are usually observed two weeks after treatment. Between the third and sixth week, most of the red marrow elements disappear, and there is central fatty infiltration in the vertebral body, or even a heterogeneous appearance pattern may be seen, resulting from the partial elimination of red marrow cellular elements. After six weeks, all patients will show hypersignal in T1. During the first year of irradiation with low doses (less than 30 Gy), there is marrow regeneration, but above 50 Gy, there is no recovery, with the MRI showing the limits between the zone of fatty infiltration and the zone of normal marrow. In case of irradiation at low doses, marrow regeneration in MRI could be confused with cellular infiltration of another type. Irradiation doses higher than 50 Gy are associated with complete replacement by fatty marrow due to irreversible marrow extinction [34].

3.3.5 Hematopoietic stem cell transplant

Knowing the normal MRI appearance of bone marrow repopulation after transplantation (BMT) is essential to be able to distinguish normal marrow repopulation from tumor infiltration. The pretransplant MRI examination may show a normal appearance of the bone marrow in the spine and pelvis or an abnormal signal corresponding to infiltration, since the examination is performed prior to myeloablative treatment. In case of obtaining an MRI in this previous phase, a tendency to decrease signal in T1 and increase in STIR is observed, a modification that may be related to cellular necrosis and bone marrow edema induced by radiation and/or chemotherapy [35].

Until the third month after allo-TMO, no changes are observed in MRI in relation to the pretransplant examination. From the sixth month onwards, the changes are due to medullary colonization after induced aplasia, with the appearance of a heterogeneous signal alternating areas of hypo- and hyperintensity in T1 or a banded appearance. This characteristic appearance observed in the vertebral bodies corresponds to cellular hypointensity in the peripheral areas below the vertebral plats and a central zone of hyperintense fatty signal. Histologically, the peripheral zones correspond to hypercellular areas of hematopoietic repopulation, while the central zone is poorly cellular and rich in fat. The distribution depends on the vascularization system of the vertebral body [36].

In addition to assessing cellularity in BMT patients, MRI can be used to study metabolic alterations derived from cytotoxic treatment or immunological processes using QSCI (chemical shift selective imaging techniques) [37].

3.3.6 Lysosomal storage diseases. Gaucher disease

In metabolic storage diseases, MRI detects the changes produced in the bone marrow due to the combination of cellular infiltration, edema, and ischemia phenomena. Cellular infiltration causes hypointense areas in T1 and T2, starting at early stages in the vertebrae (**Table 2**) and progressing from the axial to the appendicular skeleton, affecting pelvis, hips, and lower extremities [37], with proximal predominance. The typical pattern shows homogeneous signal decrease in T1 and T2 in vertebral bodies and nonhomogeneous in proximal segments of lower extremities, with preserved epiphyses in most cases.

Vascular involvement causes infarcts, avascular necrosis, and pseudosteomyelitis or bone crises. Avascular necrosis is due to chronic infarcts produced by arteriolar occlusion following progressive cellular infiltration of the marrow and episodes of vasospasm and thrombosis. In the initial phase, the marrow is isointense, and the transition between normal and necrotic tissue is a low signal band in all sequences. Subsequently, the signal of the necrotic bone decreases and fractures appear due to cortical collapse [38].

Bone infarcts are visualized as low signal foci in all sequences of intramedullary diaphyseal location and sometimes bilateral. The bone crises that appear in 30–40% of patients with Gaucher disease are caused by acute intraosseous vascular obstruction. Due to edema, the marrow appears hypointense on T1 and hyperintense on T2. Sometimes subperiosteal hyperintensity is observed on T1 due to subacute phase hematoma or hemorrhage. Control studies show recovery of the physiological signal after the episode of bone crisis.

Gaucher disease causes alterations in the vertebrae due to increased intramedullary pressure due to cellular accumulation in the form of cortical endosteal resorption and vascular occlusive phenomena. Flat vertebrae are due to necrosis and compression fractures with the widening of the disc space.

Both enzyme replacement therapy and substrate reduction therapy cause a decrease in intramedullary lipid storage already visible in some patients after six

Disease	Infiltration pattern	Diagnostic utility	Evaluation of response to treatment
Myeloma/plasmacytoma	Diffuse or focal	+++ Identify masses Global distribution Differentiate MM from MGUS	+++
Aplasia	Diffuse or mottled hyperintense in T1	++++ Assessment of residual hematopoietic foci	++++ Pattern of medullary restocking, especially in spine
Lymphoma	Diffuse or focal	Identify biopsy-approachable masses	+++
Myeloproliferative neoplasms	Diffuse or focal in mastocytosis	+ Directed biopsy in foci suggestive of mast cell accumulation	+
BMT	Normal, focal	++ Identify pretransplant marrow infiltration	+++ Pattern of normal or tumor marrow repopulation
Lysosomal storage disease. Gaucher disease	Homogeneous or heterogeneous according to localization	++++ Essential to determining the degree of BM involvement	++++ Essential to know the response rate in BM
Osteonecrosis	Hypointensity in T1 and hyperintensity in T2 due to edema	++++	++++

Table 2.
Indications for bone marrow MRI and degree of usefulness in relation to the disease.

months, with clearance and recovery of the physiological signal in MRI, as well as the disappearance of edema in bone crises [39] (**Figure 9**). In addition, in the examination of the bone marrow by MRI, other alterations not related to Gaucher disease are detected, such as vertebral hemangiomas, discopathies, etc., which stand out for their frequency in these patients [40].

3.4 Posttreatment evaluation in hematological malignancies

The initial applications of MRI in hematology were aimed at defining the presence of lesions not detectable by other imaging procedures, the maximum exponent being the assessment of intraosseous involvement in multiple myeloma. With the incorporation of BMT, MRI acquired a new dimension for the clinician, as an instrument to define the status of the BM in patients requiring this procedure, particularly in the case of bone marrow aplasia.

MRI, due to its sensitivity in the detection of cellular infiltration, is useful in the initial phase as an assessment of the extent of the disease. This quantitative extension study will also be important, together with the rest of the tests, when considering

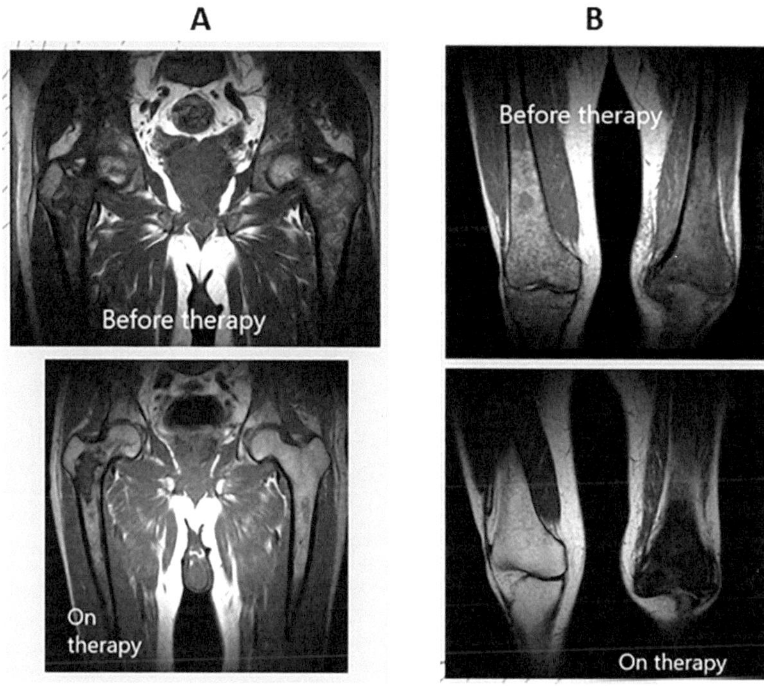

Figure 9.
Coronal spin echo (SE) T1 (A) pelvis and femurs nonhomogeneous mottled pattern with infarcts in Gaucher disease before and after therapy. The therapy causes a decrease in intramedullary lipid storage with clearance and recovery of the physiological signal. Nevertheless, complications such as infarcts or necrosis are irreversible and more visible in MRI once the infiltration has been cleared. (B) Coronal spin echo (SE) T1 femurs and tibias nonhomogeneous mottled pattern with large infarct-necrosis in Gaucher disease before and after therapy.

therapy. In the evaluation of the therapeutic response, MRI can show the degree of bone marrow involvement, being complementary to the methods that assess the progression of bone mineralization.

4. Practical considerations

MRI has proved to be a useful tool for obtaining a global map of the contents of the bone marrow cavity and the applications of the technique to the study of different processes. Assessment of bone marrow is often complex due to the presence of multiple patterns and their evolutionary change with age and disease.

Structured reports are the result of applying a logical structure to the radiological report, and the rules of elaboration comprise several criteria: (I) using a uniform language. The standardization of terminology avoids ambiguity in reporting and makes it easier to compare reports. (II) Accurately describe the radiological findings, following a prescribed order with review questions and answers. (III) Drafting using diagnostic screening tables. (IV) Respect the radiologists' workflow by facilitating the work and not hindering it [41].

The creation of structured radiological reports for the study of bone marrow is of great relevance in order to unify terms and provide the most objective assessment possible. Our group has recently published a structured report based on eight items (demographic data, diagnostic suspicion, technical data, type of exam initial or

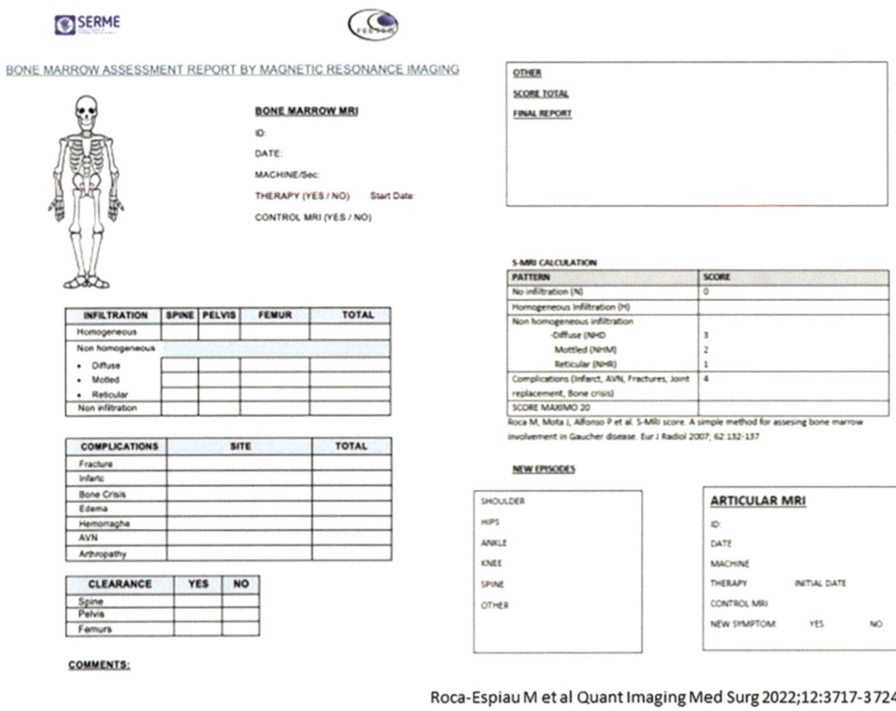

Figure 10.
Structured report for MRI bone marrow exam. Roca-Espiau et al. 2022.

control, patterns and involvement distribution, complications and their location, and summarized comments). It has been designed to provide guidance for radiologists when reporting protocol assessments to unified criteria, allow comparisons and decrease inter observers' variability [42] (**Figure 10**).

The structured radiological reports provide an answer in daily clinical practice, where situations of uncertainty are generated due to the lack of knowledge of the radiological semiology of the bone marrow, technical limitations in an extensive organ, and variability in the maturation of the bone marrow tissue and its pathological affectation. This involves both diagnosis and follow-up in the face of differentiated therapeutic approaches.

Nowadays, machine learning is revolutionizing the way data are analyzed in clinics and is helping to develop digital tools for diagnosis, disease progression prediction, and treatment responses. In our experience, using machine learning in rare diseases provides an opportunity to analyze agglomerated and heterogeneous data to create quality predictive models and identify risk features [43].

In the case of bone marrow diseases, these tools can be especially useful to speed the diagnosis and obtain better prognosis assessments and personalized care in our recently published work regarding the application of machine learning tools (random forest models) in a homogeneous Gaucher group of patients with different degrees of bone marrow infiltration and complications evaluated by MRI in order to identify features that can predict the risk of bone complications defined by the presence of intraosseous ischemic events (bone crisis, infarcts, avascular necrosis) during the follow-up. We have obtained the following information shown in **Figure 11**, model A includes all variables described as significant in a previously published study [43],

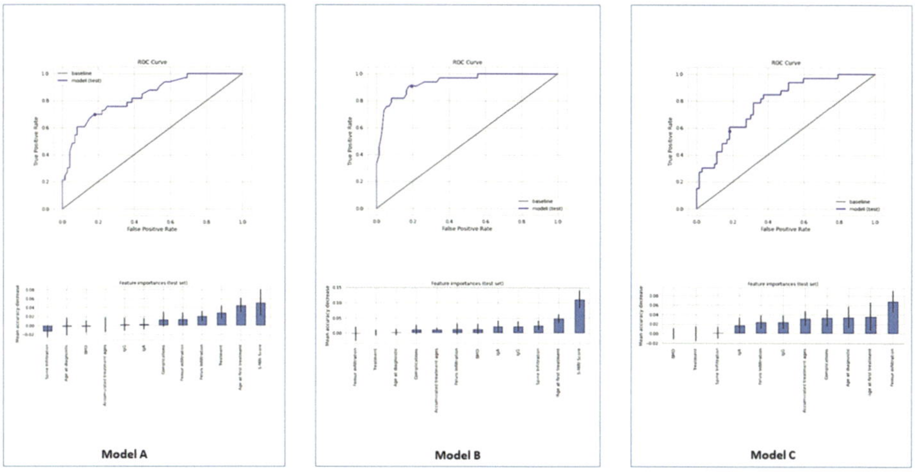

Figure 11.
ROC models. A model includes all variables. ROC B model considers whether any treatment was applied or not and features the importance of model B using the mean decrease in accuracy. ROC C model did not contain the S-MRI score and had a substantial drop in accuracy of 74.29% and an f1-score of 69.92%. The most important features for these models to predict the severity of bone affectation in Gaucher disease were the S-MRI, the age at first treatment, and the treatment used.

model B considered whether a specific treatment was applied or not, and model C ignored the degree of infiltration according to the S-MRI punctuation score [44]. The results muestran la relevancia del grado de infiltración de medulla ósea y la localización para estimar el riesgo de desarrollar complicaciones [45].

More recently, radiomics has been incorporated, which is the science of non-invasively studying features of medical images imperceptible to the human eye by applying automated algorithms to associate them with specific physiological states. Integrating clinical, biological, and therapeutic data with imaging by applying artificial intelligence methods to these studies provides a broad perspective and models that can predict the risk of complications. Today Radiomics is a science Radiomics converts medical images into mineable data by extracting quantitative characteristics [46].

The main goal is to transform imaging into actionable predictions. Programs through imaging and address healthcare issues by creating image-based predictive AI models. This outcome will allow when evaluating an MRI acquired after treatment, to assess the evolution of the patient's bone marrow involvement and to predict how they are responding to treatment. The integration of clinical, biological and/or molecular data in the classification method will be evaluated to optimize and increase its performance.

The field in which most studies are being carried out is oncology. Thanks to radiomics, diagnostic and prognostic biomarkers have been identified, associated with the development of metastases and overall patient survival in different types of cancer [47, 48].

In conclusion, in the area of bone marrow diseases, the use of machine learning provides an opportunity to analyze agglomerated and heterogeneous data to create quality predictive models and identify risk features. And it can provide important digital solutions to empower physicians to achieve health objectives [49]. Nevertheless, validation is required prior to widespread adoption in clinical practice.

Author details

Pilar Giraldo Castellano[1*] and Mercedes Roca Espiau[2]

1 Hematology, Hospital Quironsalud, FEETEG, Zaragoza, Spain

2 Radiology, FEETEG, Zaragoza, Spain

*Address all correspondence to: giraldocastellano@gmail.com

References

[1] Giraldo P, Roca M, Rubio-Félix D. Resonancia magnética en enfermedades hematológicas. Madrid: Grupo Aula Médica; 2001

[2] Liu X, Faes L, Kale AU, Wagner SK, et al. A comparison of deep learning performance against health-care professionals in detecting diseases from medical imaging: A systematic review and meta-analysis. Lancet Digital Health. 2019;**1**(6):e271-e297. DOI: 10.1016/S2589-

[3] Roca M. Resonancia magnética del sistema músculo-esquelético. Barcelona: Doyma; 1992. pp. 1-23

[4] Howe BM, Johnson GB, Wenger DE. Current concepts in MRI of focal and diffuse malignancy of bone marrow. Seminars in Musculoskeletal Radiology. 2013;**17**:137-144

[5] Vande Berg BC, Malghem J, Lecouvet FE, Maldague B. Magnetic resonance imaging of normal bone marrow. European Radiology. 1998;**8**:1327-1334

[6] Lang P, Friz R, Majumdar S, Vahlensieck M, Peterfy C, Genant HK. Hematopoietic bone marrow in the adult knee: Spin-echo and opposed-phase gradient-echo MR imaging. Skeletal Radiology. 1993;**22**:95-103

[7] Vogler JB 3rd, Murphy WA. Bone marrow imaging. Radiology. 1988;**168**(3):679-693. DOI: 10.1148/radiology.168.3.3043546

[8] Moulopoulos LA, Dimopoulos MA. Magnetic resonance imaging of the bone marrow in hematologic malignancies. Blood. 1997;**90**(6):2127-2147

[9] Roca M, Giraldo P. Magnetic resonance in the diagnosis of extent and osseous complications of Gaucher's disease type 1. Radiology (Supl.). 1997;**205**:632

[10] Bernstein ZS, Kim EB, Raje N. Bone disease in multiple myeloma: Biologic and clinical implications. Cell. 2022;**11**(15):2308. DOI: 10.3390/cells11152308

[11] Moulopoulos LA, Varma DGK, Dimopoulos MA, Leeds EN, Kim EE, Johnston DA, et al. Multiple myeloma: Spinal MR imaging in patients with untreated newly diagnosed disease. Radiology. 1992;**185**:833-840

[12] Libshitz HI, Malthouse SR, CunninghamD,MacVicarAD,HusbandJE. Multiple myeloma: Appearance at MR imaging. Radiology. 1992;**182**:833-837. DOI: 10.1148/radiology.182.3.1535904

[13] Smith DB, Scarffe JH, Eddleston B. The prognostic significance of x-ray changes at presentation and reassessment in patients with multiple myeloma. Hematological Oncology. 1998;**6**:1-6

[14] Vande Berg BC, Lecouvet FE, Michaux L, Ferrant A, Maldague B, Malghem J. Magnetic resonance imaging of the bone marrow in hematological malignancies. European Radiology. 1998;**8**:1335-1344. DOI: 10.1007/s003300050548

[15] Dimopoulos MA, Moulopoulos LA, Smith T, Delasalle KB, Alexanian R. Risk for disease progression in asymptomatic multiple myeloma. The American Journal of Medicine. 1993;**94**:57

[16] Rajkumar SV, Dimopoulos MA, Palumbo A, Blade J, Merlini G,

Mateos MV, et al. International myeloma working group updated criteria for the diagnosis of multiple myeloma. The Lancet Oncology. 2014;**15**:e538-e548

[17] Mosebach J, Thierjung H, Schlemmer HP, Delorme S. Multiple myeloma guidelines and their recent updates: Implications for imaging. Rofo. 2019;**191**(11):998-1009. DOI: 10.1055/a-0897-3966

[18] Moulopoulos LA, Dimopoulos MA, Alexanian MD, Leeds EN, Libshitz HI. Multiple myeloma: MR patterns of response to treatment. Radiology. 1994;**193**:441-446

[19] Giles SL, Messiou C, Collins DJ, Morgan VA, Simpkin CJ, West S, et al. Whole-body diffusion-weighted MR imaging for assessment of treatment response in myeloma. Radiology. 2014;**271**:785-794

[20] Baur A, Stabler A, Lamerz R, Bartl R, Reiser M. Light chain deposition disease in multiple myeloma: MR imaging features correlated with histopathological findings. Skeletal Radiology. 1988;**27**:173-176

[21] Holland J, Trenkner DA, Wasserman TH. Plasmacytoma: Treatment results and conversion to myeloma. Cancer. 1992;**69**:1513

[22] Dimopoulos M, Kyle R, Fermand JP, Rajkumar SV, San Miguel J, Chanan-Khan A, et al. International myeloma workshop consensus panel 3 - consensus recommendations for standard investigative workup: Report of the international myeloma workshop consensus panel 3. Blood. 2011;**117**:4701-4705

[23] Sanz L, Cervantes F, Mercader JM, Rozman M, Rozman C, Montserrat E. Afección oculta de la médula ósea en la enfermedad de Hodgkin: detección por resonancia magnética. Medicina Clínica. 1996;**107**:143-145

[24] Smith R, Schilder K, Shaer A, Negendak W. Lymphoma staging with bone marrow MRI. American Society of Clinical Oncology. 1995;**14**:390

[25] Albano D, Patti C, Lagalla R, Midiri M, Galia M. Whole-body MRI, FDG-PET/CT, and bone marrow biopsy, for the assessment of bone marrow involvement in patients with newly diagnosed lymphoma. Journal of Magnetic Resonance Imaging. 2017;**45**:1082-1089

[26] Resnick D, Haghighi P. Myeloproliferative disorders. In: Resnick D, editor. Diagnosis of Bone and Joint Disorders. 2.ª ed. Vol. 4. Philadelphia: Saunders; 1996

[27] Slot S, van de Donk NWCJ, Otten RHJ, Boden BJH, Zijlstra J, Raijmakers PGHM, et al. The value of bone marrow, liver, and spleen imaging in diagnosis, prognostication, and follow-up monitoring of myeloproliferative neoplasms: A systematic review. Cancer Imaging. 2021;**21**:36. DOI: 10.1186/s40644-021-00405-7

[28] Luker GD, Nguyen HM, Hoff BA, Galbán CJ, Hernando D, Chenevert TL, et al. A pilot study of quantitative MRI parametric response mapping of bone marrow fat for treatment assessment in Myelofibrosis. Tomography. 2016;**2**:67-78. DOI: 10.18383/j.tom. 2016.00115

[29] Giraldo-Castellano P, Roca-Espiau M. Exploraciones de imagen (II). In: Hernandez- Nieto L, editor. Biopsia de la médula ósea. Perspectiva clínico-patológica . 2ª ed. Madrid. 2017. pp. 193. ISBN: 978-84-697-6855-6

[30] Avila NA, Ling A, Metcalfe DD, Worobec AS. Mastocytosis: Magnetic

resonance imaging patterns of marrow disease. Skeletal Radiology. 1998;**27**:119-126

[31] Roca M, Mota J, Giraldo P, García Erce JA. Systemic mastocytosis: MRI of bone marrow involvement. European Radiology. 1999;**9**:1094-1097

[32] Marsh JC. Bone marrow failure syndromes. Clinical Medicine (London, England). 2005;**5**(4):332-336. DOI: 10.7861/clinmedicine.5-4-332

[33] Kaplan PA, Asleson RJ, Klassnen LW, Dugan MJ. Bone marrow patterns in aplastic anemia: Observations with 1.5 T MR imaging. Radiology. 1987;**164**:441-444

[34] Yang X, Bai Y, Guo H, Shi M, Zhang W, Pei Y, et al. Evaluating and monitoring bone marrow hypoplasia in adults with aplastic anemia via high-resolution iliac magnetic resonance imaging in the current era. Medicine (Baltimore). 2019;**98**(49):e18214. DOI: 10.1097/MD.0000000000018214

[35] Schick F, Einsele H, Weiss B, Jung WI, Lutz O, Claussen CD. Characterization of bone marrow after transplantation by means of magnetic resonance. Annals of Hematology. 1995;**70**:3-13. DOI: 10.1007/BF01715375

[36] Schick F, Einsele H, Weiss B, Forster J, Lutz O, Kanz L, et al. Assessment of the composition of bone marrow prior to and following autologous BMT and PBSCT by magnetic resonance. Annals of Hematology. 1996;**72**:361-370. DOI: 10.1007/s002770050187

[37] Maas M, Van Kuijk C, Stoker J, Hollak CE, Akkerman EM, Aerts JF, et al. Quantification of bone involvement in Gaucher disease: MR imaging bone marrow burden score as an alternative to Dixon quantitative chemical shift MR imaging-initial experience. Radiology. 2003;**229**:554-561

[38] Marcucci G, Zimran A, Bembi B, Kanis J, Reginster JY, Rizzoli R, et al. Gaucher disease and bone manifestations. Calcified Tissue International. 2014;**95**:477-494. DOI: 10.1007/s00223-014-9923-y

[39] Mariani G, Perri M, Minichilli F, Ortori S, Linari S, Giona F, et al. Standardization of MRI and Scintigraphic scores for assessing the severity of bone marrow involvement in adult patients with type 1 Gaucher disease. AJR. American Journal of Roentgenology. 2016;**206**:1245-1252. DOI: 10.2214/AJR.15.15294

[40] Andrade M, Valero E, Roca M, Giraldo P. The utility of magnetic resonance imaging for bone involvement in Gaucher disease. Assessing more than bone crises. Blood Cells, Molecules & Diseases. 2016;**pii: S1079-9796**(16):30219-30214

[41] Nobel JM, van Geel K, Robben SGF. Structured reporting in radiology: A systematic review to explore its potential. European Radiology. 2022;**32**:2837-2854. DOI: 10.1007/s00330-021-08327-5

[42] Roca-Espiau M, Valero-Tena E, Ereño-Ealo MJ, Giraldo P. Structured bone marrow report as an assessment tool in patients with hematopoietic disorders. Quantitative Imaging in Medicine and Surgery. 2022;**12**:3717-3724. DOI: 10.21037/qims-21-1191

[43] Andrade-Campos MM, de Frutos LL, Cebolla JJ, Serrano-Gonzalo I, Medrano-Engay B, Roca-Espiau M, et al. Identification of risk features for complication in Gaucher's disease patients: A machine learning analysis of the Spanish registry of Gaucher

disease. Orphanet Journal of Rare Diseases. 2020;**15**(1):256. DOI: 10.1186/s13023-020-01520-7

[44] Roca M, Mota J, Alfonso P, Pocoví M, Giraldo P. S-MRI score: A simple method for assessing bone marrow involvement in Gaucher disease. European Journal of Radiology. 2007;**62**:132-137. DOI: 10.1016/j.ejrad.2006.11.024

[45] Valero-Tena E, Roca-Espiau M, Verdú-Díaz J, Diaz-Manera J, Andrade-Campos M, Giraldo P. Advantages of digital technology in the assessment of bone marrow involvement in Gaucher's disease. Frontiers in Medicine (Lausanne). 12 May 2023;**10-18**:1098472. DOI: 10.3389/fmed.2023.1098472

[46] Lambin P, Leijenaar RTH, Deist TM, et al. Radiomics: The bridge between medical imaging and personalized medicine. Nature Reviews Clinical Oncology. 2017;**14**(12):749-762. DOI: 10.1038/nrclinonc.2017.141

[47] Avanzo M, Wei L, Stancanello J, Vallières M, Rao A, Morin O, et al. Machine and deep learning methods for radiomics. Medical Physics. Jun 2020;**47**(5):e185-e202. DOI: 10.1002/mp.13678

[48] Faghani S, Baffour FI, Ringler MD, Hamilton-Cave M, Rouzrokh P, Moassefi M, et al. A deep learning algorithm for detecting lytic bone lesions of multiple myeloma on CT. Skeletal Radiology. 2023;**52**(1):91-98. DOI: 10.1007/s00256-022-04160-z

[49] Jandoo T. WHO guidance for digital health: What it means for researchers. Digital Health. 2020;**6**:2055207619898984

Chapter 7

Current Topics on Knee MRI

Jorge Rolando Ortiz, Juliana Gonzalez and Juan Sebastian Herrera

Abstract

Knee pathology is one of the most common complaints worldwide. Among the most common complaints is ligamentous and meniscal injuries, for which MRI is the main diagnostic tool. Advances in MRI have improved the accuracy of detecting Anterior Cruciate Ligament (ACL), posterior cruciate ligament (PCL) and meniscal tears, which have helped orthopedic surgeons treat and classify injuries accordingly. Understanding the anatomy, different protocols and the advances will help orthopedic surgeons to deliver better patient care. MRI is especially important in ACL pathology due to its implication in femoral and tibial tunnel positioning; the more anatomically we can reconstruct the ACL, the better the functional outcomes. This is true for most of the ligamentous pathology of the knee. This chapter will review the current indication and further research areas in knee pathologies.

Keywords: ACL, posteromedial corner, posterolateral corner, postoperative meniscus, isotropic three-dimensional MRI

1. Introduction

Magnetic resonance (MR) is the preferred non-invasive imaging method to assess knee musculoskeletal injuries due to its high soft tissue resolution, and it is considered the reference standard with the additional benefit of avoiding exposition to ionizing radiation [1]. New advances in magnetic field and gradient strength allow the development of sequences for ultrastructure imaging and even postoperative ligament reconstructions or meniscal repair, which has represented a challenge to date.

Isotropic three-dimensional MR imaging has a thin slice of less than 1 mm and less partial volume artifacts with the use of thin continuous sections and oblique planes that are helpful for complex structure analysis like static and dynamic knee stabilizers with their tissue-osseous relationships [2]. These advances will be tools for preoperative planning and clinical decisions in patients with ligament and meniscal injuries.

2. Current topics in anterior cruciate ligament on MRI

The three-dimensional configuration of the anterior cruciate ligament is important to determine different conditions in association with the prognostic of the anterior cruciate ligament reconstruction, as parameters related to the most anatomical possible position. Ortiz et al. described the orientation of the anterior cruciate ligament in resonance, proposing a triplane trigonometric method; as a result, they found that the mean angle in sagittal, coronal and axial projection were 76.95, 81.65 and 33.17 degrees, respectively. It is expected that this method may be applicable for planning anterior cruciate ligament reconstruction, using the position of the anterior cruciate ligament of the uninjured knee as a reference [3].

In the evaluation of an acute lesion of the anterior cruciate ligament in MRI, there are different signs that can help with the diagnosis, the most sensitive being the discontinuity of the fibers or irregularity, increased signal on T2, bone bruises and abnormal orientation of the fibers. Secondary findings include bone lesions mainly at the level of the external femoral condyle and external tibial plateau, and it is less common to present lesions at the internal femoral condyle and tibial plateau; other findings are the anterior translation of the tibia and uncovering of the posterior horn of the lateral meniscus greater than 3.5 mm [2].

The normal appearance of the anterior cruciate ligament is characterized by a uniform caliber with a course parallel to Blumensaat's line, a high or intermediate signal on T1 and T2, and some signs of fluid between the fibers [4].

2.1 Indirect MRI signs related to anterior cruciate ligament injury

The lateral femoral notch sign is a radiographic phenomenon defined as an impaction greater than 2 mm of the lateral femoral condyle, and it may result from a traumatic episode in which the lateral femoral condyle collides with the proximal tibia, causing a defect in the lateral femoral condyle with high signal on T1 (**Figure 1**) [5, 6].

Haluk Yaka validated a posterior base measurement of the medial and lateral meniscus, defined as a line passing through the tibial edge of the meniscus and a line passing through the capsular edge on the sagittal side of the posterior horn of the meniscus based on the previous studies performed by Hohman where the relation of the posterior angle of the base of the meniscus and its relationship with the anterior cruciate ligament injury was discussed, it was concluded that the medial and lateral angles above 84.5 and 93.15, respectively are an indirect finding of anterior cruciate ligament injury (**Figure 2**) [7].

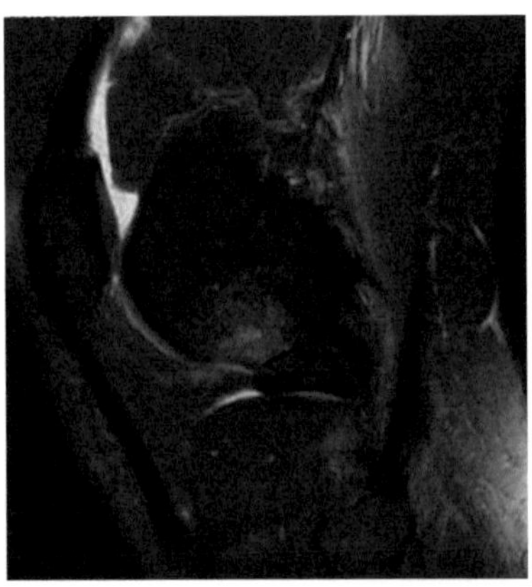

Figure 1.
Lateral Femoral Condylar Notch, Indirect Sign of Anterior Cruciate Ligament Injury.

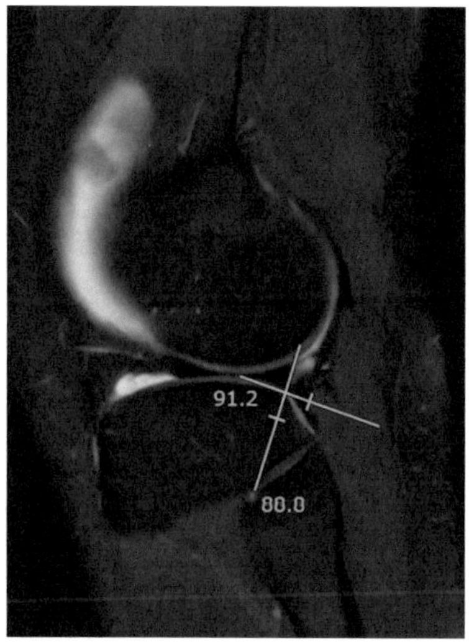

Figure 2.
Posterior base meniscus angle, a line through the base of the meniscus and a line through de posterior aspect of the meniscus in the sagittal plane.

2.2 Location of anterior cruciate ligament injury point in MRI

Within the management protocol for anterior cruciate ligament injuries, there is the option of performing primary repair in cases in which the injury is proximal near the insertion of the femur and a contained injury with good tissue. In order to validate this condition, Sherman classified injuries into five types, been I and II types the proximal tears, in which a primary ACL repair can be considered. Now, before performing an arthroscopy, it is important to know if the patient is a candidate for repair or not; it could change the treatment and rehabilitation approach. For this purpose, it has been described in recent years to resonance as a method that allows us to know the location of the rupture of the anterior cruciate ligament [8, 9].

In a study carried out by Guillien et al. at the University of Rennes, they evaluated the correlation between the anterior cruciate ligament lesion point determined in MRI in comparison with the findings in arthroscopy, and this study was based on the Sherman classification (**Figure 3**). It was identified that the correlation in relation to the position of the lesion is approximately 70%; it was not the same for the evaluation of the quality of the ligament determined in resonance, in which the correlation was 50%. In another work carried out by Vanderlist, the predictive capacity of preoperative resonance is evaluated in relation to anterior cruciate ligament repair in Sherman type I and II injuries, finding that in 90% of the cases that a lesion was diagnosed pre-surgical type I repair of the ACL was performed and in 88% of type II [4].

As mentioned previously, the complex three-dimensional ACL orientation does not allow for the complete visualization of the ligament in a single image. ACL runs obliquely through the intercondylar notch; this is why various MRI techniques including oblique planes have been investigated (**Figure 4**) [3].

Kwon et al. from the Department of Radiology and Center for Imaging Science and Department of Orthopedic Surgery of Samsung Medical Center, Seoul, Korea, published a study whose purpose was to evaluate the diagnostic role of additional use of oblique coronal and oblique sagittal imaging for an ACL injury [10]. The study

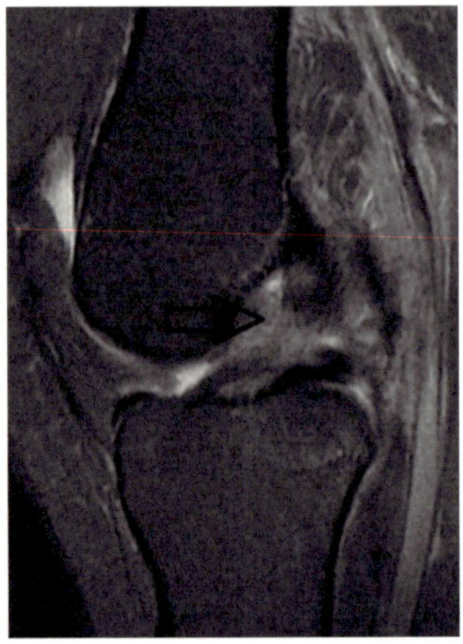

Figure 3.
Anterior cruciate ligament tear in the proximal third of the ligament.

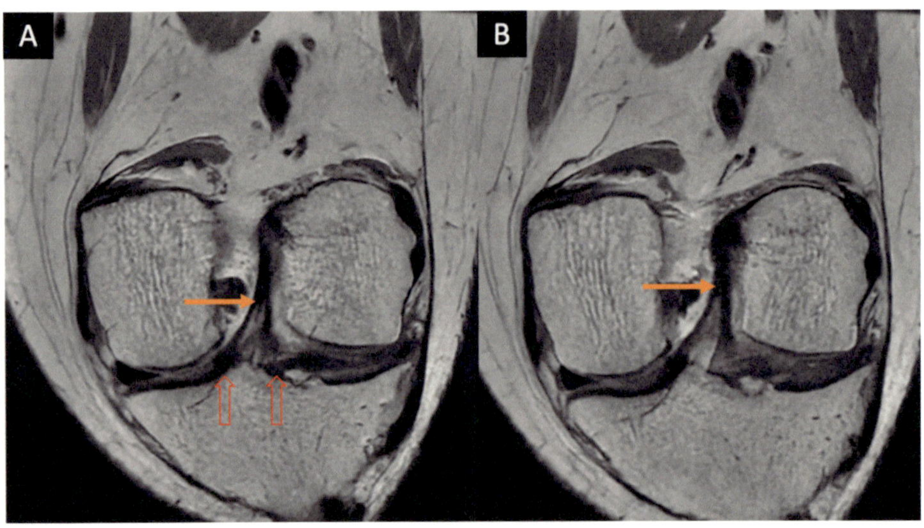

Figure 4.
A 55-year-old female left knee. Oblique coronal PD FSE MR images, performed using a 1.5 T system with 1.2 mm thickness (A) anterior bundles of ACL (arrow) and it is possible evaluate posterior meniscal roots (red open arrows). (B) Posterior bundles of ACL (arrow).

population consisted of 101 patients with a mean age of 35 +/− 12.6 years who required knee arthroscopy for suspected of having a torn ACL on MRI examination with both orthogonal and oblique images using 1.5 MRI system conventional protocol sequences with section thickness 3 mm, TR/TE 2000–3800/20-30 ms and additional oblique coronal/sagittal proton density-weighted imaging. The oblique sagittal image was made in the plane parallel to the medial border of the lateral femoral condyle on an orthogonal coronal image and the oblique coronal image was obtained in plane parallel to course of the femoral intercondylar roof using a sagittal image. Two musculoskeletal radiologists analyzed the knees MRI retrospectively, without knowledge about arthroscopic results, then determined intact, probable tear or definite ACL tear. They evaluated sequences by using four methods (*M*), *MA*: orthogonal images only, *MB*: orthogonal and oblique coronal, *MC*: orthogonal and oblique sagittal, and *MD*: orthogonal, oblique coronal and sagittal images.

Diagnostic performance with sensitivities, specificities and accuracies of each method respect arthroscopy (partial or complete ACL tear) as a gold standard was as follows respectively, MA 95%, 83.6%, 88.1%, MB 97.5%, 95.1%, 96%, MC 97.5%, 95.1%, 96% and MD 97.5%, 98.4%, 98%, meaning that specificities and accuracies for methods B, C D were statistically significantly higher than method A. No difference was found between methods B, C and D. This study concludes that some oblique imaging added to standard MRI sequences improves the ability to diagnose ACL tears [10].

2.3 Mucoid degeneration of the anterior cruciate ligament

A topic of interest in recent years has been mucoid degeneration of the anterior cruciate ligament as a rare entity, which can be confused with an ACL lesion, being difficult to diagnose. Bergins et al. described an incidence of 1.8% in an analysis of 4221 patients, in addition to describing different aspects that can help diagnose mucoid degeneration of the anterior cruciate ligament, which includes the presence of a uniform thickening with a bulging ligament, semiologically described as "celery stalk," increased intermediate intraligamentary signal on T1, and hyperintensity on T2, maintaining orientation and continuity of the anterior cruciate ligament fibers. More recently, Cilengir et al. described MRI findings that can help differentiate mucoid degeneration of the anterior cruciate ligament from injury and found an increased prevalence of intraosseous femoral cysts being part of the mucoid degeneration. Other authors have described anatomical conditions in resonance that can be associated with mucoid degeneration of the anterior cruciate ligament, such as an increase in the angle of the tibial slope, a decrease in the width of the intercondylar groove, male sex [11–13].

3. MRI accuracy of posterolateral and posteromedial corners injuries

3.1 Normal anatomy of the posterolateral corner

Posterolateral corner (PLC) is currently a diagnostic challenge.

PLC structures are grouped into primary stabilizers, which are statics, and secondary stabilizers, which are static and dynamic [14]. PLC structures are the main mechanism to protect against knee varus stress and posterolateral rotation of the tibia with respect to the femur [15–17].

Table 1 shows all the PLC structures with their respective origins and insertions, and the graphic scheme of the structures is shown in **Figure 5**.

The three primary stabilizers are the fibular collateral ligament (FCL), popliteus tendon (PLT) and popliteofibular ligament (PFL). FCL is the main stabilizer with varus stress, and PLT acts as a stabilizer regarding tibial external rotation.

On magnetic resonance (MR) imaging FCL is visualized on axial and coronal plane as low signal-intensity band extending from the lateral epicondyle to the lateral aspect of the proximal fibula. The PLT is seen as a low-signal-intensity structure on axial or sagittal sequences [18].

Structure	Origin	Insertion
Fibular collateral ligament	Small bony depression proximal and posterior to the lateral epincondyle	Fibular head distal to the tip of the fibular styloid.
Popliteus tendon	From popliteus sulcus of the lateral femoral condyle	Runs posteromedially deep to the fibular collateral ligament, exits the joint capsule through the popliteus hiatus and inserts along the posteromedial aspect of the proximal tibia.
Popliteofibular ligament	From popliteus tendon proximal to the myotendinous junction	Inserts onto the medial downslope of the fibular styloid.
Midthird lateral capsular ligament	Thickening of the lateral capsule from the lateral epicondyle of the femur	Capsular attachments to the lateral meniscus and inserts onto the tibia anterior to popliteal hiatus
Popliteomeniscal fascicles	Popliteus tendon	Posterior horn of the lateral meniscus
Lateral gastrocnemius tendon	Posterior lateral femoral condyle	Achilles tendon onto calcaneus
Fabellofibular ligament	Thickened distal aspect of the biceps femoris that extends from an osseous fabella (sesamoid bone)	Fibular styloid.
Arcuate ligament	Y-shaped thickening of the posterolateral join capsule	Fibular styloid with the fabellofibular ligament
Biceps femoris	Ischiatic tuberosity and femoral diaphysis	Consists of a long and short head and also has numerous insertions arms on fibular styloid and tibial lateral condyle
Iliotibial band	It is a thick band of fascia formed proximally at the hip by the fascia of the gluteus maximus, gluteus medius and tensor fasciae latae muscles.	Gerdy's tubercle

Table 1.
Components of the posterolateral corner.

The PFL has an anterior and posterior bundle that embraces the popliteus myotendinous junction, and it is best seen as a low-T2-signal structure on coronal and sagittal planes, deep to the inferior lateral genicular vessels. However, the PFL is not currently described in conventional MR imaging. Coronal oblique sequences and isotropic 3D MR improve visualization of these tissues (**Figure 6**) [19, 20].

Secondary stabilizers include the mid-third lateral capsular ligament (ALT), popliteomeniscal fascicles (PMF), lateral gastrocnemius tendon (LG), fabellofibular ligament (FFL), arcuate ligament, biceps femoris tendon and iliotibial band.

The ALT that is a thickening of the lateral capsule of the knee is seen on isotropic 3D MR axial images [20].

The popliteomeniscal fascicles form the roof and floor of the popliteus hiatus. They are visible in 60–94% of patients and can be seen on sagittal images of isotropic 3D MR.

FFL is best seen on sagittal and coronal MR imaging posterior to the lateral inferior genicular artery; however, this ligament is visible in 33–48% of patients.

Arcuate ligament is also inconsistent, but it may be identified as a thin band overlying the PLT on axial sequences [20].

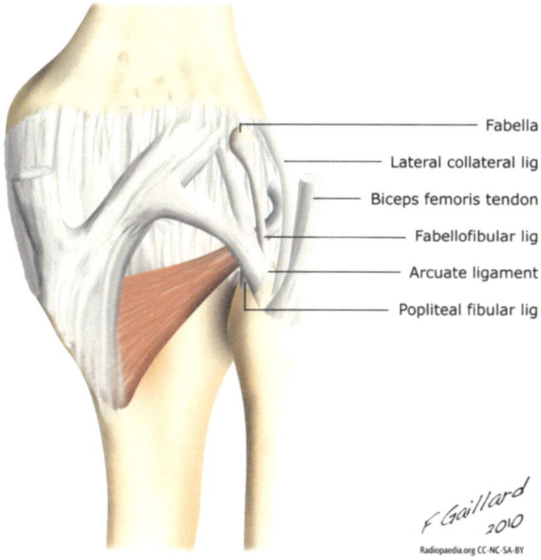

Figure 5.
Scheme of the structures of the posterolateral corner.

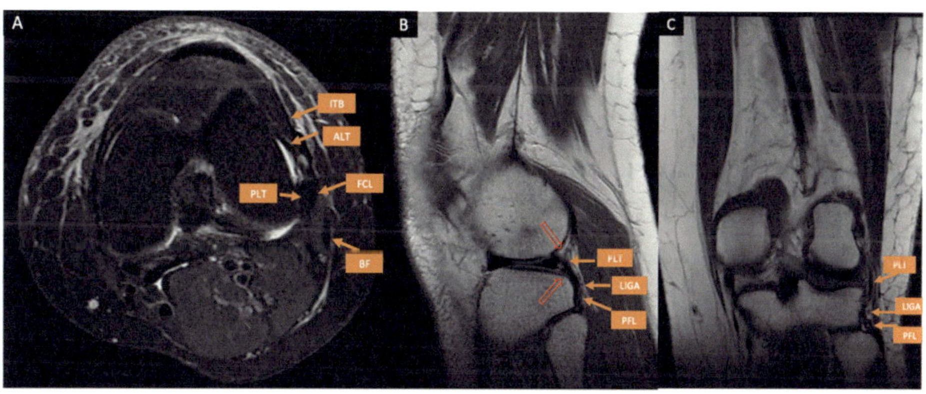

Figure 6.
MR images of a left knee of a 40-years old female patient. (A) Axial fat-saturated T2 weighted sequence demonstrates posterolateral structures. Popliteus tendon (PLT), fibular collateral ligament (FCL), biceps femoris tendon (BF), lateral capsular ligament (ALT), iliotibial band (ITB). (B) Sagittal proton density-weighted image lateral knee with popliteus hiatus formed by popliteomeniscal fascicles (red open arrows) and Popliteofibular ligament (PFL) located anterior to lateral inferior genicular artery (LIGA). (C) Coronal T1 image that shows PFL and its association with respect to LIGA.

Biceps femoris tendon (BFT) is composed of multiple distal insertion arms that may not be easily distinguishable but just long and short arms (**Figure 6**).

3.2 Posterolateral corner injuries and MR imaging

Injuries to the PLC most commonly occur with varus forces, particularly to a hyperextended knee or associated with knee dislocation. Diagnosis may be difficult in the setting of acute trauma because of the patient's joint effusion. However, prompt diagnosis and management are important, as unrecognized PLC injuries may result in chronic instability and premature osteoarthritis [21]. Therefore, it would be desirable to predict not only by clinical testing but also by imaging. **Figure** 7 shows PLC injury patterns on MR imaging.

A meta-analysis established that 1.5-T or 3.0-T MRI offers high diagnostic accuracy for evaluating injuries involving the meniscus, anterior cruciate and posterior cruciate ligaments. However, in multi-ligament injured knees, MRI had been found to have lower accuracy for the detection of PLC ligament tears [22].

A recent retrospective study from the Ottawa Hospital Research Institute and Department of Radiology determined the diagnostic performance of preoperative MRI for diagnosing PLC injuries of patients with knee dislocations compared to intraoperative findings [21]. They included 39 patients who required repair/reconstruction of the posterolateral corner between May 2005 and April 2020. Preoperative MRI of these patients was on 1.5 T or 3.0 T scanners, and all protocols included sequences in standard imaging planes.

The fibular collateral ligament, bicep femoris and popliteus tendon were categorized as normal, partial tear or complete tear. The posterolateral ligamento-capsule complex (LCC) was evaluated as a single unit that includes popliteofibular and fabellofibular ligaments. This complex and posterolateral capsule was classified as intact or torn; the same classification was used for intraoperative findings.

The *diagnostic performance* of MRI was a sensitivity (Se) of 95% and specificity (Sp) of 100% for detecting fibular collateral ligament (FCL) tears, Se of 100% and Sp of 77% for BFT tears, Se of 88% and Sp of 71% for PLT injuries and Se of 97% and Sp of 33% for LCC tears. The correlation between surgical findings and magnetic resonance of PLC structures was strongest for the BFT and weakest for the LCC.

This study reports accuracy ranging from 82 to 95% for detecting PLC injuries with MR imaging, even higher than other previous studies [23], probably associated with MRI evolution in the last few years.

Longer time between injury and surgery may allow some injuries to heal and can be found intact at surgery but still presenting with abnormal signals at MRI, leading to higher false positive counts; obtaining MR images closer to the time of injury may

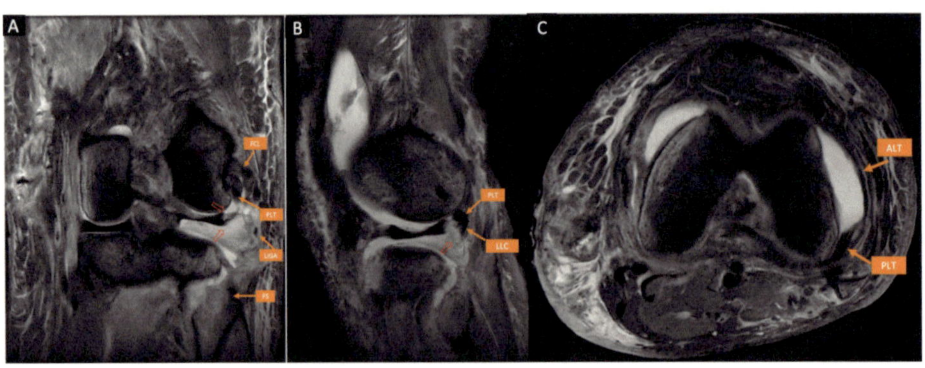

Figure 7.
MR images of a 23-year-old man with left knee PLC injury caused in a motorcycle accident. (A) Coronal proton-density weighted fat-saturated T2 sequence with popliteomeniscal fascicles disruption (red open arrow) and complete tear of fibular collateral ligament (FCL) and popliteus tendon (PLT). Lateral inferior genicular artery (LIGA), fibular styloid (FS). (B) Sagittal proton-density weighted fat-saturated T2 image with PLT tear and disruption of posterolateral ligamento-capsule complex (LCC) and evident disruption of poplitemeniscal fascicles (red open arrow). (C) Axial proton-density weighted fat-saturated T2 sequence with posterolateral capsule injury, midthird lateral capsular ligament (ALT).

make their interpretation more challenging due to inflammatory process also affecting the radiologist reading [24].

Finally, this study concludes that despite the challenges of evaluating knee posterolateral corners, MRI has an acceptable accuracy for detecting their injuries.

Statistically, up to 20% of MRIs made in patients with an Anterior Cruciate Ligament (ACL) tear may reveal PLC injuries. A Swiss retrospective cohort study of The University of Zurich determined the diagnostic performance of different MR imaging findings for helping to predict posterolateral instability in patients with acute complete ACL tears by performing a decision tree analysis [25]. Their sample comprises 162 patients who underwent ACL reconstruction with or without concomitant posterolateral corner reconstruction. Clinical diagnosis of PLC instability requiring reconstruction served as gold standard, and there were obtained conventional MRI of all patients. Results demonstrated a low sensitivity and high specificity for posterior cruciate ligament, biceps femoris, popliteus tendon and lateral collateral ligament. Decision tree analysis results showed that a complete tear or fibular avulsion of the FCL was the most statistically significant finding to help predict posterolateral instability. These results are shared with other studies that affirm it is sufficient to assess the FCL, BFT and PLT to predict PLC instability [26].

With respect to small structures, this study confirms variable visibility of popliteofibular ligament, fabellofibular ligament and popliteomeniscal fascicles, which are not always observed at conventional two-dimensional MRI.

Limitations of this study are sample of patients limited to ACL reconstruction, MRI performed in the acute trauma 10 days or less, and it was different protocol and scanners to take images like in many other studies.

In the next years, the use of isotropic three-dimensional high-resolution sequences could allow for oblique reconstructions and individual examination for each patient. A retrospective study performed at Gachon University of South Korea aimed to document the appearance of PLC structures on 3D isotropic and routine two-dimensional MR images and to determine the significance of pathologic findings in patients with confirmed posterolateral instability. They evaluate conventional 3.0 T MRI of 25 patients with surgery indication as the gold standard and also of 25 control patients with any radiological or clinical finding, but in addition to standard sequences 3D isotropic SPACE (Sampling perfection with Application optimized Contrasts using different flip angle Evolution) images were obtained until adequate visualization of posterolateral corner. Their findings were the following:

- The popliteofibular ligament was best seen with 3D isotropic images. The lateral geniculate artery appeared as a landmark.
- 3D images detected normal and partial tears (grade 1 or 3) of PLC, and 2D images just when there were complete tears (grade 4).
- The "fibular cap sing" that represents no-osseous avulsion of the distal FCL from the tip of the proximal fibula on 3D images was found to be useful for the diagnosis of PLC tears.

A disadvantage of 3D isotropic imaging is the lack of fat suppression that may underestimate slightly altered ligament signals.

Despite these limitations, 3D isotropic SPACE MRI could be an interesting examination method in institutes interested in multiligamentary knee reconstruction [26].

3.3 Normal anatomy of the posteromedial corner

The posteromedial corner (PMC) contains the structures lying between the posterior margin of the superficial medial collateral ligament (MCL) and the medial border of the posterior cruciate ligament (PCL). These structures avoid anteromedial rotational instability and provide restraint to valgus stress. Although some authors do not consider MCL to be part of posteromedial corner, recently, an international expert consensus panel has included it [27, 28]. **Figure 8** illustrates the borders of the PMC, **Table 2** shows PMC structures with their respective origins and insertions, and **Table 3**, **Figures 9** and **10** describe normal MR imaging of PMC.

3.4 Posteromedial corner injuries and MR imaging

The semimembranosus is the main dynamic stabilizer of the PMC; without its dynamic support, the remaining PMC structures fail over time and lead to instability that affects the anterior cruciate ligament or posterior cruciate ligament [32].

MR imaging is the modality of choice for PMC injury assessment; however, at present, there are no specific studies that have evaluated the sensitivity and specificity of PMC structure injuries on MR imaging, unlike PLC structures.

A retrospective study of patients with symptomatic anteromedial rotational instability who were treated with ligament reconstruction and based on surgical descriptions found injury of the posterior oblique ligament (POL) in 99% of the cases, injury to the semimembranosus in 70% and peripheral meniscal detachment in 30% [33].

Tears in these three structures are well defined on MRI with an established classification system for each one of the ligament structure injuries.

House et al. have proposed the same classification used for the MCL injuries in the POL injuries, and it is grade I, intact ligament with edema surrounding it (T2

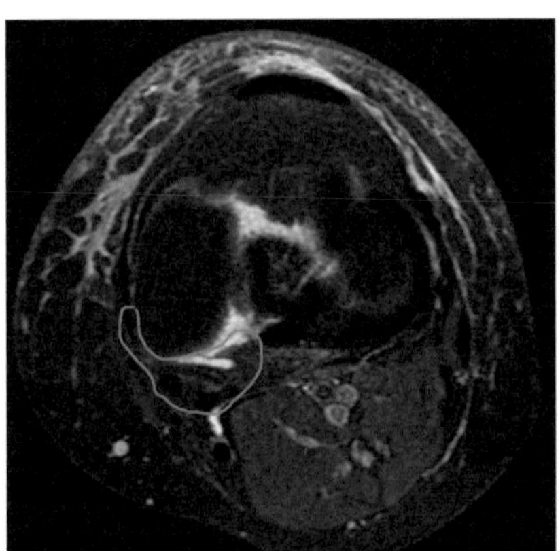

Figure 8.
Axial fat-saturated MR image of a left knee illustrated the borders of the PMC (green outline).

Structure	Origin	Insertion
Semimebranosus tendon	Ischiatic tuberosity	5 expansions • Direct arm (principal attachment) • Capsular arm • Extension to the OPL • Anterior arm or reflected arm • Inferior or popliteal arm
Oblique Popliteal Ligament (OPL)	Arises from the capsular arm of the POL and lateral expansion of the semimembranosus	Attaches to fabella, the meniscofemoral portion of the posterolateral joint capsule and plantaris muscle.
Posterior oblique ligament (POL)	Origin distal and posterior to adductor tubercle	3 arms in the posteromedial aspect of medial meniscus and the tibia. • Central or tibial arm • Superior or capsular arm • Distal arm
Posteromedial capsule	Includes deep MCL with its meniscotibial and meniscofemoral components	It is reinforced externally by the POL and expansions from the semimembranosus
Posterior horn of the medial meniscus	Posterior horn has a "Brake stop" function to anterior translation of the tibia	The medial meniscus attaches to the capsule posteromedially and the meniscotibial ligament anchors the meniscus to the tibia

Table 2.
Components of the posteromedial corner.

Structure	MR Imaging
Semimebranosus tendon **Figure** 7, **Figure** 8	• Direct arm is seen in sagittal and axial images along the posteromedial aspect of the tibia distal to the articular margin • Anterior arm is seen on coronal plane as an oval structure deep to the MCL • Other expansions are difficult to identify [29, 30]
Oblique Popliteal Ligament (OPL) **Figure** 7, **Figure** 8	The OPL is a thin structure and is difficult to distinguish from the posterior joint capsule. When is thicker, it is seen on sequential sagittal and axial images as a band extending obliquely from the main tendon of semimembranosus laterally toward lateral femoral condyle [27].
Posterior oblique ligament (POL) **Figure** 7, **Figure** 8	POL is best visualized on coronal and axial images at the level of the femoral condyle. The three arms run continuously with each other, are difficult to distinguish from each other [30, 31].
Posteromedial capsule	The attachment of the peripheral surface of the meniscus to the capsule and the tibia is best evaluated on sequential coronal and sagittal images posterior to the superficial MCL [30].
Medial collateral ligament **Figure** 7, **Figure** 8	Best visualized on coronal and axial images.

Table 3.
Normal MR imaging of PMC structures.

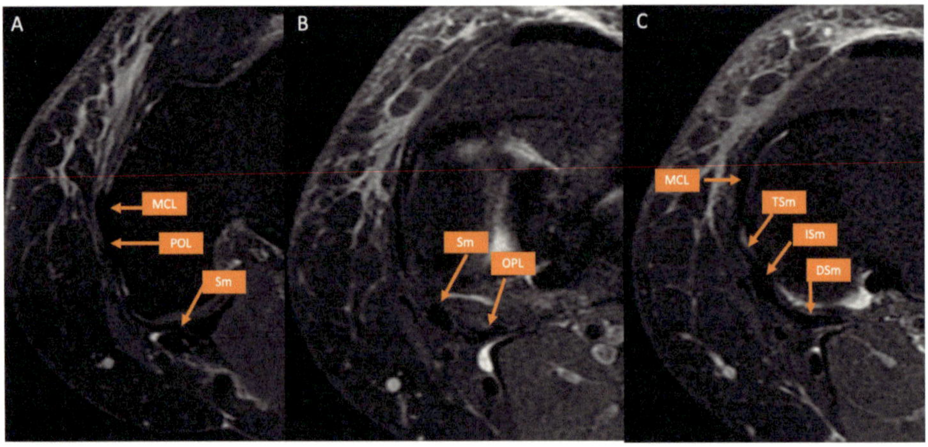

Figure 9.
Axial proton density weighted fat-saturated MR images of a normal knee, proximal to distal. (A) At the level of the femoral condyles illustrates medial collateral ligament (MCL), posterior oblique ligament (POL) and semimembranosus tendon (Sm). (B) At the level of joint space, oblique popliteal ligament (OPL). (C) At tibial plateau level, tibial semimembranosus expansion (TSm), inferior arm (ISm) and direct arm (DSm).

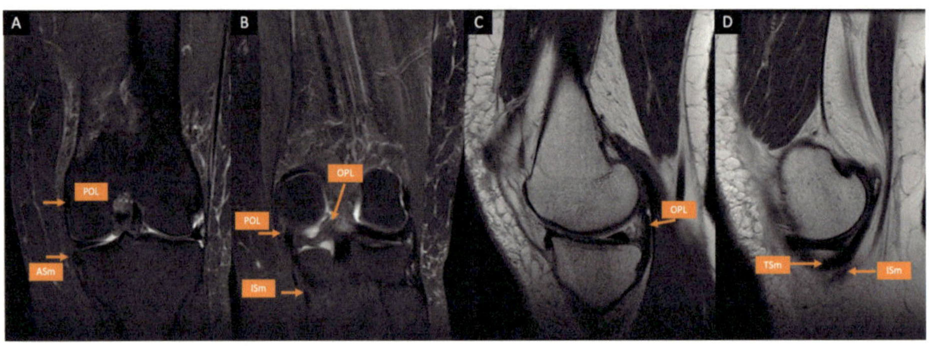

Figure 10.
Coronal proton-density weighted fat-saturated images and sagittal proton density images of a normal left knee. (A) Posterior oblique ligament (POL), anterior expansion of semimembranosus (ASm). (B) Inferior semimembranosus arm (ISm). (C) Oblique popliteal ligament (OPL), (D) Tibial and inferior expansions of semimembranosus.

high signal). Grade II thickening of the ligament with partial disruption of fibers and Grade III with complete disruption of the ligament [34]. The coronal plane allowed for visualization of the POL; however, the coronal oblique plane, in combination with the axial plane, improved the analysis of the POL. In case of doubt, the addition of intraarticular contrast material can optimize the visualization of the POL and capsular layers in the axial plane as these structures are displaced away from the femur (**Figure 11**) [35].

With respect to medial meniscocapsular injuries, a "reverse Segond fracture" represents meniscotibial ligament osseous avulsion, also associated with posterior cruciate ligament rupture. Meniscocapsular separation is best visualized in the sagittal sequences. When there is increased signal intensity and thickening of the capsule, it may

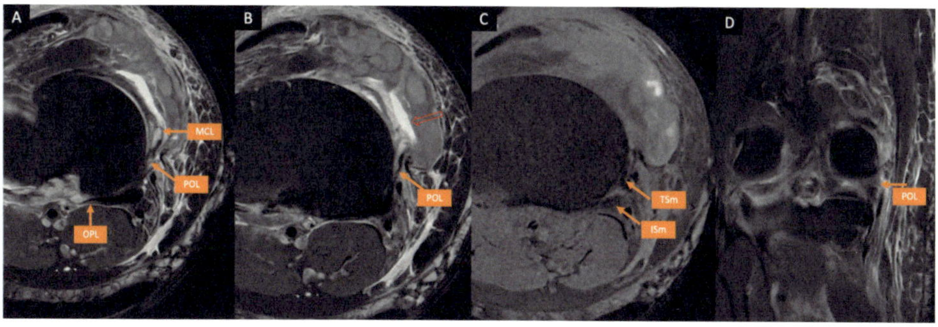

Figure 11.
MRI of a 53-year-old man with right knee PMC injury caused in a twisting knee injury. (A) (B) axial proton density weighted fat-saturated sequence at the level of joint space and at tibial plateau level respectively illustrate OPL partial tear, POL, MCL complete tears and capsular separation (red open arrow). (C) Axial T1 fat-saturated image shows tibial (TSm) and inferior (ISm) semimembranosus arms injuries. (D) Coronal proton-density weighted fat-saturated image with POL complete tear.

be associated with capsule sprain, but it could be a ruptured popliteal cyst, too. Hence, it is important to interpret according to clinical history and other imaging features.

4. MR imaging of the postoperative meniscus

Meniscal surgery is a frequent orthopedic procedure [36]. Clinical examination and MR imaging are both the current way to assess patients who complaint about knee pain after meniscectomy or meniscus repair. However, the evaluation after surgery can be difficult and represents a challenge to date.

The normal medial and lateral meniscus are hypointense on T1- and T2-weighted MR images. On axial plane, they are like C-shape; on sagittal images, they appear as a wedge configuration; on coronal plane, they are seen as a right-triangular with a free edge oriented to intercondylar notch [37–39].

Sagittal and coronal images of intermediate and/or T1-weightened sequences of conventional MRI are the method of choice to assess signal changes in nonoperative meniscus, however after meniscal surgical procedure, it is the T2-to-intermediate-weighted fluid-sensitive images in sagittal and coronal planes to detect synovial fluid signal extending into the substance of the meniscus indicating that the articular surface has been breached due to a new retear [39].

In regard to magnetic resonance with contrast, direct magnetic resonance arthrography (MRA) is useful to evaluate recurrent tears or unhealed repair when there is an extension of contrast into a meniscus substance. Disadvantages of this examination include other invasive procedures, infection, bleeding and allergic reactions. If there is fluoroscopic-guided injection, radiation exposure is another risk and finally entails more costs. In some countries, it is considered an off-label use of gadolinium-based contrast agents, according to FDA [40].

Indirect MR arthrography involves the intravenous administration of gadolinium-based contrast; it allows the identification of sites of hyperemic synovitis associated with vascular tissue enhancement. Nevertheless, the stable healed granulation tissue, as expected after meniscus surgery, may be difficult to differentiate from a residual tear, and it may result in potential false positives. Disadvantages are costs, patient time and adverse reaction to contrast agents [40].

4.1 Imaging findings after meniscectomy

Low signal linear fibrotic tissue in Hoffa fat pad is. A sign of precious arthroscopic knee surgery [39, 40]. With respect to partial or total meniscectomy, it could be found:

Diminution of meniscal tissue, ranging from a large portion of the meniscus being removed to mild blunting of the apical margin [39].

Baker et al. reviewed PubMed published evidence from 1990 to 2017 about recurrent tears after partial meniscectomy imaging. They found nine studies that reported the accuracy of conventional MRI, direct MRA and indirect MR arthrography compared to second-look arthroscopy. Conventional MRI had accuracy ranging from 57 to 80%, direct MRA from 85 to 93% and indirect MRA from 81 to 93% [40]. However, some other studies, specifically a randomized cohort study made by White et al., published in Radiology Journal compare the accuracy of conventional MRI, direct MRA and indirect MRA, with inconclusive results that do not find statistical differences among the three techniques in the setting of a recurrent meniscal tear, although there was a trend toward increased diagnostic performance for both direct and indirect MRA [41].

Intermediate-signal intensity extending to the articular surface of the postoperative meniscus on fluid-sensitive sequences has been the most specific sign of retear [41], meaning that its absence could be a negative predictive sign of an intact meniscus after surgery (**Figure 12**) [39, 42].

4.2 MRI findings after meniscal repair surgery

In this kind of surgery, intrinsic high signal may be seen on intermediate and T2 MRI such as the features of preoperative meniscal injury.

A cohort study performed by the Institute of Sports Medicine of Peking University evaluated the diagnostic performance of MRI compared with second-look arthroscopy as the gold standard in 81 patients to evaluate the healing of the repaired meniscus. They found T2-weighted sagittal and coronal sequences had higher specificity (89.6–98.7%, respectively) and accuracy (85.4–91%), while T1 and proton density had higher sensitivity, 91.7% and 75%-83–3%, respectively. The diagnostic value could be improved by a combined application of different sequences [43].

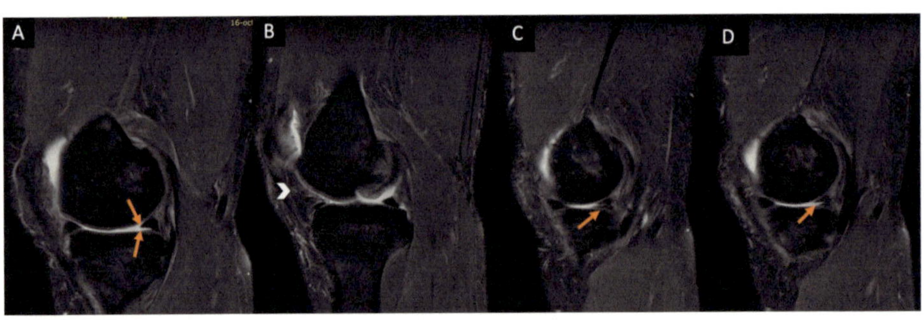

Figure 12.
(A) A 62-year-old man following partial medial meniscectomy, sagittal fat-saturated T2 and sagittal proton density images respectively that show diminutive body and posterior horn of medial meniscus (orange arrows) and (B) fibrotic stranding in Hoffa fat pad (arrowhead). (C) and (B) same patient. Sagittal fat-saturated T2-weighted image illustrates surfacing intermediate signal extending to the apical meniscal articular surface characteristic of a new tear.

The same study by Pekin University also demonstrated that approximately 50% of the patients with intact menisci in diagnostic arthroscopy illustrating features of surfacing increased intermediate-weighted linear signal at the healed repair site [43].

On MRA, one of the findings that may represent a partially healed repair or a partial thickness recurrent tear is the extension of intraarticular contrast through the meniscal repair site from one articular surface to another [39].

As a clinical care point, MRI or direct and indirect MR arthrography is the examination of choice for patients with suspected meniscus retear. However, those methods can be challenging because conventional diagnostic criteria of a meniscal tear may be normal findings postoperatively.

5. Three-dimensional isotropic MRI of radial and root tear of meniscus

Almost all meniscal injuries have suggested that the sagittal imaging sequences are the most accurate for detecting them; however, the radial and the root tears could be missed on conventional 2D images due to thicker slices of axial sequences, which is the preferred plane to evaluate both. Several studies describe thin-Section 3D FSE sequences such as Volume isotropic turbo spin echo acquisition (VISTA), CUBE and SPACE to analyze menisci injuries with better quality image of peripheral and radial tears (**Figure 13**) [44].

Daekeon Lim et al. from Yonsei University College of Medicine, Seoul, Korea, assessed the diagnostic value of FS 3D VISTA (*Volume isotropic turbo spin echo acquisition*) protocol imaging compared to 2D standard imaging in detecting arthroscopy-confirmed (gold standard) radial and root tears. Their results reported sensitivity and specificity of 96% and 96% with VISTA protocol imaging, respectively, versus 87% and 91% with 2D imaging. They found higher sensitivity and specificity with isotropic 3D imaging and excellent interobserver agreement for detecting meniscal radial and root tears. Some limitations and bias were retrospective study design, size

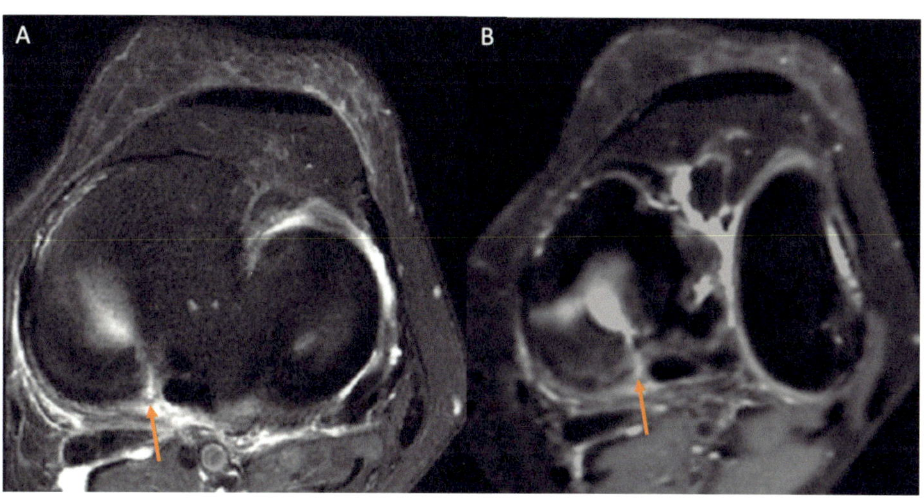

Figure 13.
A 45-year-old female left knee. MRI were performed using a 3.0 T system with 2 mm thickness (A) PD FSE FS axial 2D image with suspected tear of posterior root of medial meniscus (arrow). (B) Multiplanar reformatted axial 3D VISTA (volume isotropic turbo spin echo acquisition) image of 0.5 mm slice thickness with better delineation of posterior root tear (arrow).

of sample, and MRI readers were aware that patients had undergone arthroscopic surgery that could overestimate the lesions [44].

6. Conclusions

The advances in magnetic resonance research imaging have made it possible to achieve greater detail in the diagnosis of knee joint pathologies. Different protocols and MRI sequences have been described, as well as clinical signs for different conditions such as posterolateral corner lesions and mucoid degeneration of the anterior cruciate ligament. These tools should be used as part of the clinical approach to patients with traumatic knee injuries.

Conflict of interest

The authors declare no conflict of interest.

Author details

Jorge Rolando Ortiz[1,2*†], Juliana Gonzalez[1†] and Juan Sebastian Herrera[1†]

1 Department of Trauma and Orthopedics, Universidad Nacional de Colombia, Colombia

2 Hospital Universitario Nacional de Colombia, Colombia

*Address all correspondence to: jrortizmo@unal.edu.co

† These authors contributed equally.

References

[1] Zhao M, Zhou Y, Chang J, Hu J, Liu H, Wang S, et al. The accuracy of MRI in the diagnosis of anterior cruciate ligament injury. Annals of Translational Medicine. 2020;**8**(24):1657-1657. DOI: 10.21037/atm-20-7391

[2] Chhabra A, Ashikyan O, Hlis R, Cai A, Planchard K, Xi Y, et al. The International Society of Arthroscopy, knee surgery and orthopaedic sports medicine classification of knee meniscus tears: Three-dimensional MRI and arthroscopy correlation. European Radiology. 2019;**29**(11):6372-6384. DOI: 10.1007/s00330-019-06220-w

[3] Morales JRO, López L, Herrera JS, Martínez JT, Buitrago G. Three-dimensional orientation of the native anterior cruciate ligament in magnetic resonance imaging. The Journal of Knee Surgery. 2023;**36**(14):1438-1446. DOI: 10.1055/a-1946-6143

[4] Mehier C, Ract I, Metten MA, Najihi N, Guillin R. Primary anterior cruciate ligament repair: Magnetic resonance imaging characterisation of reparable lesions and correlation with arthroscopy. European Radiology. 2022;**32**(1):582-592. DOI: 10.1007/s00330-021-08155-7

[5] Lucidi GA, Grassi A, Di Paolo S, Agostinone P, Neri MP, Macchiarola L, et al. The lateral femoral notch sign is correlated with increased rotatory laxity after anterior cruciate ligament injury: Pivot shift quantification with a surgical navigation system. American Journal of Sports Medicine. 2021;**49**(3):649-655. DOI: 10.1177/0363546519876648

[6] Bernholt D, DePhillipo NN, Aman ZS, Samuelsen BT, Kennedy MI, LaPrade RF. Increased posterior tibial slope results in increased incidence of posterior lateral meniscal root tears in ACL reconstruction patients. Knee Surgery, Sports Traumatology, Arthroscopy. 2021;**29**(11):3883-3891. DOI: 10.1007/s00167-021-06456-4

[7] Yaka H, Türkmen F, Özer M. A new indirect magnetic resonance imaging finding in anterior cruciate ligament injuries: Medial and lateral meniscus posterior base angle Haluk Yaka. Joint Diseases and Related Surgery. 2022;**33**(2):399-405. DOI: 10.52312/jdrs.2022.653

[8] Jog AV, Smith TJ, Pipitone PS, Toorkey BC, Morgan CD, Bartolozzi AR. Is a partial anterior cruciate ligament tear truly partial? A clinical, arthroscopic, and histologic investigation. Arthroscopy: The Journal of Arthroscopic and Related Surgery. 2020;**36**(6):1706-1713. DOI: 10.1016/j.arthro.2020.02.037

[9] Van der List JP, DiFelice GS. Preoperative magnetic resonance imaging predicts eligibility for arthroscopic primary anterior cruciate ligament repair. Knee Surgery, Sports Traumatology, Arthroscopy. 2018;**26**(2):660-671. DOI: 10.1007/s00167-017-4646-z

[10] Kwon JW, Yoon YC, Kim YN, Ahn JH, Choe BK. Which oblique plane is more hepful in diagnosing an anterior cruciate ligament tear. Clinical Radiology. 2009;**54**:291-297. DOI: 10.1016/j.crad.2008.10.007

[11] Sasaki R, Nagashima M, Takeshima K, Otani T, Okada Y, Aida S, et al. Association between magnetic resonance imaging characteristics and pathological findings in entire

posterior cruciate ligament with mucoid degeneration. Journal of International Medical Research. 2022;**50**(3):1-10. DOI: 10.1177/03000605221084865

[12] Hotchen AJ, Demetriou C, Edwards D, JTK M. Mucoid degeneration of the anterior cruciate ligament: Characterization of natural history, femoral notch width index, and patient reported outcome measures. The Journal of Knee Surgery. Georg Thieme Verlag. 2019;**32**:577-583. DOI: 10.1055/s-0038-1660514

[13] Kaya A, Köken M, Akan B, Karagüven D, Güçlü B. The triangle between the anterior and posterior cruciate ligaments: An arthroscopic anatomy study. Acta Orthopaedica et Traumatologica Turcica. 2015;**49**(5):478-482. DOI: 10.3944/AOTT.2015.14.0402

[14] LaPrade RF, Ly TV, Wentorf FA. The posterolateral attachments of the knee: A qualitative and quantitative morphologic analysis of the fibular collateral ligament, popliteus tendon, popliteofibular ligament, and lateral gastrocnemius tendon. The American Journal of Sports Medicine. 2003;**31**(6):854-860. DOI: 10.1177/03635465030310062101

[15] LaPrade RF, Tso A, Wentorf FA. Force measurements on the fibular collateral ligaments, popliteofibular ligament and popliteus tendon to applied loads. The American Journal of Sports Medicine. 2004;**32**(7):1695-1701. DOI: 10.1177/0363546503262694

[16] Grood ES, Stowers SF, Noyes FR. Limits of movement in the human knee. Effect of sectioning the posterior cruciate ligament and posterolateral structures. The Journal of Bone and Joint Surgery. American Volume. 1988;**70**(1):88-97

[17] LaPrade RF, Wozniczka JK, Stellmaker MP. Analysis of the static function of the popliteus tendon and evaluation of an anatomic reconstruction: The "fifth ligament" of the knee. The American Journal of Sports Medicine. 2010;**38**(3):543-549. DOI: 10.1177/0363546509349493

[18] Rosas HG. Unraveling the posterolateral corner of the knee. Radiographics. 2016;**36**(6):1776-1791. DOI: 10.1148/rg.2016160027

[19] Rajeswaran G, Lee JC, Healy JC. MRI of the popliteofibular ligament: Isotropic 3D WE-DESS versus coronal oblique fat-suppressed T2W MRI. Skeletal Radiology. 2007;**36**(12):1141-1146. DOI: 10.1007/s00256-007-0385-4

[20] Khodarahmi I, Alizai H, Alaia E, Gyftopoulos S. MR imaging of the knee posterolateral and posteromedial corner injuries. Magnetic Resonance Imaging Clinics of North America. 2022;**30**:215-226. DOI: 10.1016/j.mric.2021.11.003

[21] Rakhra K, Delorme JP, Sanders B, Liew A. The diagnostic accuracy of MRE for evaluating the posterolateral corner in acute knee dislocation. European Radiology. 2022;**32**:6752-6758. DOI: 10.1007/s00330-022-08986-y

[22] Cheng Q, Zhao FC. Comparing of 1.5- and 3.0-T magnetic resonance imaging for evaluating lesions of the knee A systematic review and meta-analysis (PRISMA-compliant article). Medicine. 2018;**98**(38):1-9. DOI: 10.1097/MD.0000000000012401

[23] Twaddle BC, Hunter JC, Chapman JR, Simonian PT, Escobedo EM. MRI in acute knee dislocation. A prospective study of clinical, MRI, and surgical findings. Journal of Bone and Joint Surgery. British Volume (London). 1996;**78**:573-579

[24] Rubin DA, Kettering JM, Towers JD, Britton CA. MR imaging of knees having

isolated and combine ligament injuries. American Journal of Roentgenology. 1998;**170**:1207-1213. DOI: 10.2214/ajr.170.5.9574586

[25] Filli L, Rosskopf A, Sutter R, Fucentese S, Pfirrmann C. MRI predictor of posterolateral corner instability: A decision tree analysis of patients with acute anterior cruciate ligament tear. Radiology. 2018;**00**:1-11. DOI: 10.1148/radiol.2018180194

[26] Collins MS, Bond JR, Crush AB, Stuart MJ, King AH, Levy BA. MRI injury patterns in surgically confirmed and reconstructed posterolateral corner knee injuries. Knee Surgery, Sports Traumatology, Arthroscopy. 2015;**23**(10):2943-2949. DOI: 10.1007/s00167-015-3738-x

[27] Lundquist RB, Matcuk GR, Schein AJ, Skalski MR, White EA, Forrester DM, et al. Posteromedial corner of the knee: The neglected corner. Radiographics. 2015;**35**:1123-1137. DOI: 10.1148/rg.2015140166

[28] Chahla J, Kunze KN, Laprade RF. The posteromedial corner of the of the knee: An international expert consensus statement on diagnosis, classification, treatment and rehabilitation. Knee Surgery, Sports Traumatology, Arthroscopy. 2020;**29**(9):2976-2986. DOI: 10.1007/s00167-020-06336-3

[29] Benninger B, Delamarter T. Distal semimembranosus muscle-tendon-unit review: Morphology, accurate terminology, and clinical relevance. Folia Morphologica. 2013;**72**(1):1-9. DOI: 10.5603/fm.2013.0001

[30] De Maeseneer M, Shahabpour M, Lenchik L. Distal insertions of the semimembranosus tendon: MR imaging with anatomic correlation. Skeletal Radiology. 2014;**43**(6):413-432. DOI: 10.1007/s00256-014-1830-9

[31] Beltran J, Matityahu A, Hwang K. The distal semimembranosus complex: Normal MR anatomy, variants, biomechanics and pathology. Skeletal Radiology. 2003;**32**(8):435-445. DOI: 10.1007/s00256-003-0641-1

[32] Geiger D, Chang E, Pathria M, Chung CB. Posterolateral and posteromedial corner injuries of the knee. Radiologic Clinics of North America. 2013;**51**(3):413-432. DOI: 10.1016/j.rcl.2012.10.004

[33] Sims FW, Jacobson KE. The posteromedial corner of the knee medial-sided injury patterns revisited. The American Journal of Sports Medicine. 2004;**32**(2):337-345. DOI: 10.1177/0363546503261738

[34] House CV, Connell DA, Saifuddin A. Posteromedial corner injuries of the knee. Clinical Radiology. 2007;**62**:539-546. DOI: 10.1016/j.crad.2006.11.024

[35] D'Ambrosi R, Corona K, Guerra G, Cerciello S, Chiara U, Ursino N, et al. Posterior oblique ligament of the knee: State of the art. EFORT Open Reviews. 2021;**6**:364-371. DOI: 10.1302/2058-5241.6.200127

[36] Montgomery SR, Zhang A, Ngo SS. Cross-sectional analysis of trends in meniscectomy and meniscus repair. Orthopedics. 2013;**36**(8):1007-1013. DOI: 10.3928/01477447-20130724-15

[37] Robson MD, Gatehouse PD, Bydder M. Magnetic resonance: An introduction to ultrashort TE (UTE) imaging. Journal of Computer Assisted Tomography. 2003;**27**(6):825-846. DOI:10.1097/00004728-200311000-00001

[38] Nguyen JC, De Smet AA, Graf BK. MR imaging-based diagnosis and classification of meniscal tears. Radiographics. 2014;**34**(4):981-999. DOI: 10.1148/rg.344125202

[39] Fierstra S, Lawrence MW. MR imaging of the postoperative meniscus. Magnetic Resonance Imaging Clinics of North America. 2022;**30**:351-362. DOI: 10.1016/j.mric.2021.11.012

[40] Baker JC, Friedman MV, Rubin DA. Imaging the postoperative knee meniscus: An evidence-based review. AJR. American Journal of Roentgenology. 2018;**211**(3):519-527. DOI: 10.2214/AJR.18.19692

[41] White LM, Schweitzer ME, Weishaupt D. Diagnosis of recurrent meniscal tears: Diagnosis of recurrent meniscal tears: Prospective evaluation of conventional MR imaging, indirect MR arthrography and direct MR arthrography. Radiology. 2002;**222**(2):421-429. DOI: 10.1148/radiol.2222010396

[42] Kijowski R, Rosas H, Williams A. MRI characteristics of torn and untorn post-operative menisci. Skeletal Radiology. 2017;**46**(10):1353-1360. DOI: 10.1007/s00256-017-2695-5

[43] Miao Y, Yu JK, Ao YF, Zheng ZZ, Gong X, Ming Leung KK. Diagnostic values of 3 methods for evaluating meniscal healing status after meniscal repair. Comparison among second-look arthroscopy, clinical assessment, and magnetic resonance imaging. The American Journal of Sports Medicine. 2011;**39**(4):735-742. DOI: 10.1177/0363546510388930

[44] Lim D, Han Lee Y, Kim S, Song HT, Suh JS. Fat-suppressed volume isotropic turbo spin echo acquisition (VISTA) MR imaging in evaluating radial and root tears of the meniscus: Focusing on reader-defined axial reconstruction. European Journal of Radiology. 2013;**82**:2296-2302. DOI: 10.1016/j.ejrad.2013.08.013

Chapter 8

Magnetic Resonance Imaging Pulse Sequence Selection for Optimal Time and Image Quality Enhancement

Naima Amin and Muhammad Yousaf

Abstract

This study is a comparison of three commonly used magnetic resonance imaging (MRI) pulse sequences to examine the image quality of the pulse sequences at a short acquisition time. Two tissue-equivalent gels were created. While one gel is constructed of polysaccharide and agarose, the other is made of ferrous benzoic xylenol orange (FBX). FBX gel is exposed to a 25 Grey dosage of 6MV photons from a linear accelerator. Repetition time (TR) was used to conduct experimental modifications in imaging parameters. The quantitative analysis comprises the signal-to-noise ratio (SNR) and contrast-to-noise ratio (CNR). Fast Spin Echo (FSE) and Fast Fluid Attenuated Inversion Recovery (FLAIR) are most comparable in SNR at 1.5 Tesla for various TR values. Conventional Spin Echo (CSE) has a CNR that is 143% and 93% higher than FSE and FLAIR, respectively. The time difference between CSE and FSE is 6 minutes and 34 seconds, whereas CSE and FLAIR is 6 minutes and 43 seconds. FSE and FLAIR provide superior image quality with quicker acquisition, suitable for patients sensitive to longer scan durations. Meanwhile, CSE stands out, delivering significantly enhanced contrast and SNR in T2-weighted images compared to other MRI pulses.

Keywords: acquisition time, pulse sequences, magnetic resonance imaging, repetition time, signal to noise ratio, contrast to noise ratio

1. Introduction

1.1 Magnetic resonance imaging

An extremely versatile, noninvasive medical imaging method that produces high-quality images is magnetic resonance imaging (MRI). It opposed to ionising imaging techniques like X-ray CT. For image development, MRI does not use ionising radiation. It is a sophisticated diagnostic tool that offers precise anatomical information, good spatial resolution and strong cellular comparison. The sensitivity of MR signals to a variety of tissue factors allows for the acquisition of detailed information. MRI is the best imaging method for evaluating the cerebrum/skull, and **cardiovascular** activities, in addition to the digestive organs, blood vessels, skeletal system, and abdomen because of its outstanding soft-tissue contrast [1, 2].

1.2 Image quality of MRI

Image quality is a parameter used to assess the diagnostic efficacy and interpretation of an image. The selection of the pulse sequence in MRI impacts the weighting and quality of the image, as well as its ability to respond to disorders. It is critical to understand these parameters and their interplay in order to achieve the best image quality [3]. Signal-to-noise ratio (SNR), the amount of pixels used to create an image in digital form, and difference between living organism tissue are the primary MRI picture quality and diagnostic factors for human tissues. All of these elements are interconnected and subject to the fundamental principles of NMR physics, it is difficult for them to improve at the same time. New developments in the field of MRI technology have resulted in increases in contrast and SNR through the modification of imaging parameters required. Many factors influence the MRI image quality. It is crucial to understand these aspects, how they interact, and how to get the best possible image quality. The image quality is primarily affected by four elements, which are

- Signal to noise ratio
- Contrast to noise ratio
- Image Homogeneity
- Scan time

1.3 Signal to noise ratio

The difference between the received signal's amplitude and the noise's average amplitude is known as the signal to noise ratio. The recipient coil generates a voltage that produces a signal as the NMV (nuclear magnetic vector) moves in a circular motion within the transverse plane.

Frequencies that randomly arrange themselves in space and time give rise to noises. Background electrical noise from the system and the patient's presence in the magnet combined to create unnecessary noise in an MR environment. The presence of the patient in the MRI, the area being investigated, and the system's inherent noise all contribute to this noise, which is constant for every patient. SNR increases and better images are produced when the signal gets comparatively shorter than the noise.

The SNR plays a key role in determining the clinical MRI quality; hence having the maximum SNR is necessary to avoid having a poor image quality.

1.4 Contrast to noise ratio

The comparative difference in signal intensity between two adjacent portions of a picture is also defined as contrast of the picture.

CNR quantifies the distinguishability or contrast between these regions, taking into account the noise level in the image. Contrast refers to the basic difference or distinction in the luminescence of each pixel within an image in the framework of MRI, which is determined by the intensity of the signal received from each voxel during the NMR experiment.

Variations in the spin relaxation velocities are the primary cause of the differences in signal intensity. Additionally, the hydrogen density of the tissues varies and is crucial for contrast discrimination.

MRI is a highly valuable technique for assessing oncological conditions because it offers exceptional contrast in soft tissues. By utilising a variety of pulse sequences that produce different contrasts, detailed evaluations of the disease's size and extent can be conducted.

1.5 Image homogeneity

Image uniformity reflects how evenly the signal intensity is distributed across the image. A high level of image homogeneity is desirable as it ensures that the MR system is accurately capturing the underlying properties of the imaged object. Homogeneity is particularly important in clinical MRI to provide reliable and consistent image quality, aiding in accurate diagnosis and interpretation of the images. Factors such as magnetic field uniformity, scanner calibration, and appropriate. A common artefact in MR imaging, known by various names such as intensity non-uniformity, bias, inhomogeneity, or shading artefact, can impact the constancy of MR signal intensity.

To maximise clinical outcomes, it is important to understand the impact of changing the imaging parameters of an MR pulse sequence. The quality of an image, or MR intensity non-uniformity, is greatly influenced by the repetition time (TR) and number of echoes.

1.6 MRI scan time

MRI is a widely utilised technique for obtaining highly detailed images of various objects, such as the human body. The total scan time refers to the duration required to gather all the necessary data for generating the desired images or to complete the K-space filling process.

Longer scan times increase the patient's likelihood of moving during the acquisition, which is critical for maintaining image quality. Any patient movement during the scan may cause the images to be compromised. However, extended acquisition times have the disadvantage of lowering image quality due to a number of artefacts, including respiratory artefacts. Reducing scan time in Magnetic Resonance Imaging (MRI) continues to be a crucial concern, particularly in clinical settings where diagnostic images need to be obtained. Acquiring images of excellent quality in a short period of time is crucial for optimising the diagnostic technique.

1.7 Acquisition time issues of MRI

Although MRI is a more accurate and non-invasive medical tool for clinical diagnosis, its lengthy acquisition time reduces its patient comfort and significance [4]. The duration of the MRI scan is crucial for maintaining image quality. Any patient movement during the scan could potentially result in blurry images [5]. However, one consequence of a long acquisition period [6] is that image quality reduction due to a variety of artefacts, including respiratory artefacts [7, 8].

Every advanced pulse sequence due to fast acquisition time possesses some negative aspect. Parallel imaging loses SNR and could result in technique-dependent artefacts, however it is a successful method for reducing scan times [9]. There is an inverse correlation between the speed of image acquisition and total image quality [10].

The available options for pulse sequences and acquisition factors are incredibly extensive and patient compliance is an issue with the selection of acquisition parameters [11]. Reducing the duration of MRI scans remains a significant challenge, especially when considering the acquisition of diagnostic images within a clinical setting [12].

Maintaining the image quality, i.e., contrast to noise ratio, signal to noise ratio and image uniformity, is crucial when selecting quick acquisition pulse sequences. Each pulse sequence performs differently as a result of its unique properties and attributes [13].

In MRI, increasing the value of TR results in longer acquisition durations for T2-weighted images. It is critical to gather high-quality images quickly in order to ensure an optimal diagnostic strategy [14]. The scan duration should always be as short as possible to minimise the possibility of patient movement.

A variety of approaches can be used to increase the quality of clinical information gained from an MR image. To analyse and choose the best technique for a certain organ, comparisons between various pulse sequences are always done. In order to evaluate the best imaging procedure for an MRI of a very short T2, in 2016, Ali Caglar Ozen and colleagues compared MRI of an ancient mummified human hand using an ultra-short echo time sequence [15]. To examine the effectiveness of widely used soft tissue suppression techniques on a quantitative level, Chang Li in 2012 compared optimised soft tissue suppression schemes for ultrashort echo time MRI [16]. Michael P. Recht increases the value of MRI by reengineering the MRI workflow to reduce MRI acquisition time [17].

1.8 Purpose of the comparison of MRI pulse sequences

The aim of this study is to evaluate and compare the commonly employed pulse sequences used at the clinical level. The purpose is to determine their performance and select the most appropriate pulse sequence based on factors such as SNR, CNR, and collection time, specifically for T2-weighted images. The optimum image quality at a quick acquisition time would be achieved with a continuous range of TR. Additionally; the effectiveness of the traditional spin echo sequence in the presence of various quick pulse sequences was examined in the present investigation. Fast Fluid Attenuated Inversion Recovery (FLAIR), Conventional Spin Echo (CSE), and Fast Spin Echo (FSE) were the three pulse sequences that were used the most frequently in the present study.

2. Phantom preparation

2.1 First gel

A polysaccharide gel along with agarose is used in an experiment at Ninewells Hospital and Medical School in Dundee, UK, to create a substance that is similar to tissue for MRI. For imaging applications, this substance contains gadolinium chloride attached to ethylene diamine tetraacetic acid (EDTA). The T1 and T2 values of this substance may differ, independently as a result of varying the proportions of each ingredient.

When creating a substance that is an equivalent to biological tissue, the gadolinium ions are chelated to the macromolecule EDTA, which has three distinct benefits.

First, the chelation takes away any chance that the ions will engage in any further chemical reactions with the gel matrix. Second, chelation may prevent the hydroxyl ions from being released by the gadolinium ions. The chelation procedure moderately affects the Gd-EDTA solution's empirical relaxing characteristics. This effect, however, becomes more pronounced at higher frequencies, notably above 30 MHz [18].

This work employs seven 12 mm diameter phantoms. For those phantoms, the T1/T2 intervals of relaxation are 608/134, 759/155, 917/135, 986/220, 1050/164, 1180/221, and 1296/200 (msec). The 1.5 T unit (Siemens MAGNETOM Avanto, UK) is used for MR imaging (**Figure 1**). A 1.5 mm region of interest (ROI) was cantered in the gel for estimating signal intensity and replicating the ROI to measure the signal intensity of the background noise. SNRs have been determined with the following equation.

$$SNR = SI/N \quad (1)$$

Where N is the surrounding standard error of variance and SI is the mean magnitude of the signal of the ROI situated in the middle of the gel. SNR was examined using software called Image J. Phantom scanning uses the CP Head Coil of the MRI. Certain imaging parameters of CSE, FSE, and FLAIR were constant throughout the investigation, comprising the following parameters: the entire amount of acquisitions (1), the proportion of sampling (100), the field of view (100 mm x100 mm), the pixel per mm resolution (1.280), and the segment width (4 mm). Furthermore, the FSE pulse sequence had a consistent inversion time of 860 ms and an echo train length of 5, whereas the FLAIR pulse sequence had a constant inversion time of 860 ms and an echo train length of 5.

The outcomes of our evaluation were assessed using the practical information provided by the MHRA (Medicine and Healthcare Products Regulatory Agency) Evaluation 04133 for the Siemens Magetom Avanto 1.5 T system [19]. The percentage error indicates the discrepancy between the value that was observed and the actual

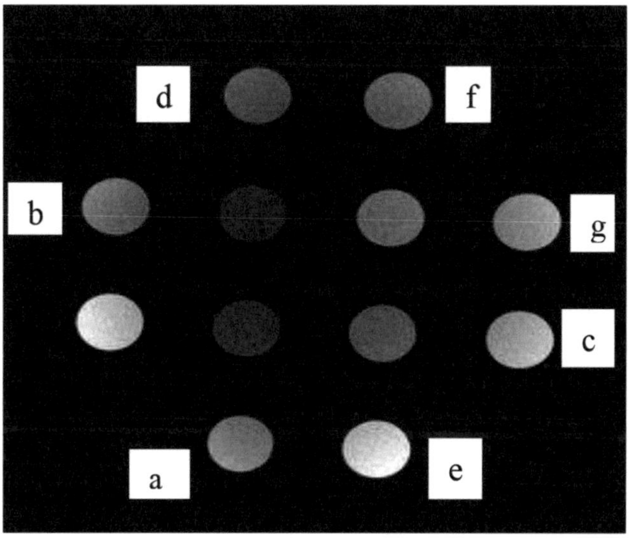

Figure 1.
Polysaccharide, comprise the range of relaxation value for biological tissues at Siemens MAGNETOM Avanto 1.5 T.

value. Using MATLAB 7.7 (R2008b), the curve fitting approach is used to approximate the optimised value.

Gelatine (from bovine skin, Type B), sulphuric acid (Sigma-Aldrich), Xylenol Orange Tetrasodium salt (Sigma-Aldrich), and Benzoic Acid (Sigma-Aldrich) were used to make the second gel, Ferrous Benzoic Xylenol Orange (FBX), which was developed in 1998 by Kelly RG [20] alongside other researchers [21–23].

2.2 Second gel

A one-litre capacity container was used to combine 5 ml of benzoic acid, 1 ml of Xylenol Orange, and 25 ml of sulphuric acid to create the stock solution, which was then left to sit at room temperature. The first step in creating gel is to mix 40 g of gelatine with 700 ml of distilled water, 25 ml of sulphuric acid, and a hot plate that has been prepared to 40°C. After stirring continuously for 30 minutes, the gel's gelatine melted. 0.1 mm of ferrous sulphate was dissolved in 100 ml of Xylenol vibrant orange base solution with benzoic acid. The resulting solution was then added to the liquid gelatin. By adding 25 ml of the solution, a gel with a final volume of 1 litre was created. The preliminary oxygen concentrations in the solution affect how the Fricke gel dosimeter responds. During preparation, the gel is exposed to the air, and six test containers with a 10 ml capacity are used to pour the gel into for the irradiation of different doses. At 5°C, all gel phantoms were kept [24].

2.3 Gel irradiated and MRI scanning

Radiation was applied to the gel using a 6MV photon beam generated by a Varian Clinic 600C Linear accelerator. The dose was 25GY delivered at a Source to Surface Distance (SSD) of 95.5 cm with a field area of 55 cm^2. Siemens MAGNETOM Avanto, a 1.5 T machine, is used to perform MR imaging. Phantom scanning uses the CP body Coil of the MRI. The CSE, FSE, and FLAIR pulse sequences were used to image the phantom (**Figure 2**).

A 1.5 mm square ROI was set in the gel's middle to analyse signal intensities for quantitative image processing. The same ROI area was used to measure noise within the background. This process is performed throughout each pulse sequence. The following formula is used to determine contrast to noise ratios (CNRs):

$$CNR = SNR_A - SNR_B \tag{2}$$

The phantom's contrast to noise ratio of exposed to radiation and non-exposed to radiation regions is denoted by SNR_A and SNR_B, respectively.

For the T2-weighted investigation, imaging parameters for CSE, FSE, and FLAIR are kept constant (100 x 100 mm field of view; 4 mm slice thickness). The number of acquisitions was 1; for the T2-weighted study, the FLAIR inversion time was 2500 ms; the length of the echo train was 21; and for the FSE, the echo train length was 21.

2.4 T1/T2 calculation of FXG gel with variation of deliver dose

The same methods used by Afzal et al. [25, 26], Bartusek et al. [20, 27], and MATLAB version (R2008b) are utilised to calculate T1/T2 for FGX Gel (**Table 1**).

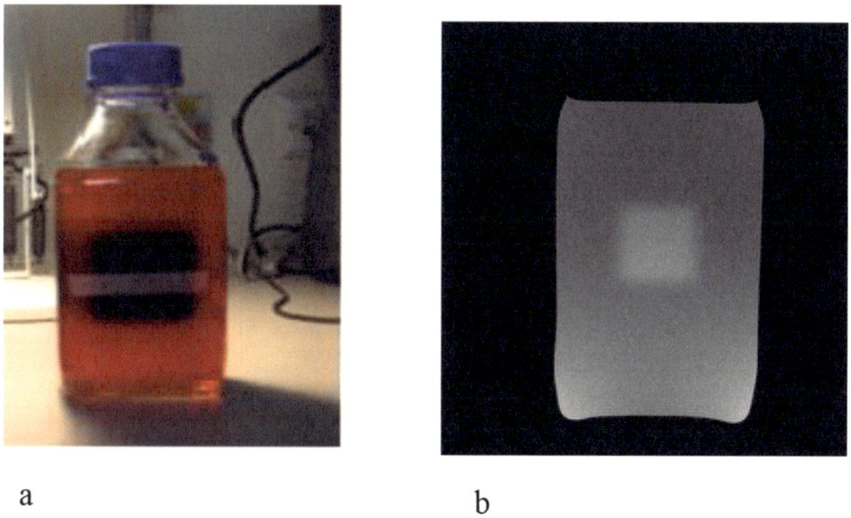

Figure 2.
FXG phantom (a) after irradiation; deliver dose is 25 Grey with linear accelerator, 600 MV X-ray energy (b) MR image of FGX phantom in CSE.

Dose	T1 (msec)	T2 (msec)
O Grey (No dose)	812	166
25 Grey	628	58

Table 1.
Calculated values of FGX at 0 gray and 25 gray.

3. Analysis of CSE, FSE, and FLAIR responses for SNR and CNR for various phantoms and parameters

The T2-weighted images and prolonged acquisition time made CSE less noteworthy compared to other pulse sequences. Both CSE and FLAIR generate the necessary SNR, but FLAIR has an advantage because to its quick acquisition time, as seen in **Table 2**, T1/T2 time of the phantom is 608/134 (msec). For accurate SNR of the image, FLAIR takes 56% less time to acquire than CSE (**Figure 3a**).

The minimum TR value in **Table 3**, the phantom's T1/T2 time is 759/155 (msec), CSE is the one that best MRI technique that satisfies the SNR requirement. FSE or FLAIR, on the other hand, can be considered better pulse sequences due to their fast acquisition times. For achieving an appropriate SNR of the image, the FSE and FLAIR pulse sequences were found to take 79% and 80% less time, respectively, compared to the CSE sequence (**Figure 3b**).

As demonstrated in **Table 4**, only CSE produces SNR for images with a minimal TR. T1/T2 is 917/135 (msec) for the phantom. The significance of other pulse sequences is diminished for this particular phantom due to inadequate SNR (**Figure 3c**).

CSE and FSE both are present in the significant domain of SNR, as seen in **Table 5**; T1/T2 time for that phantom is 986/220 (msec) while the faster acquisition time of

Sr. no	Pulse sequences	T1/T2 of phantom (msec)	TR (msec)	SNR	Percentage error (%)	Acquisition time (min: sec)
1	CSE	608/134	1800	130.23	−11.40	5.9
			2000	140.72	−4.27	6.29
			2200	146.83		7.08
			2400	149.44		8.59
2	FSE	608/134	4000	127.52	−13.24	0.48
			4200	133.44	−9.22	1.29
			4400	139.02	−5.42	1.5
			4600	160.33	2.12	2.18
3	FLAIR	608/134	4000	128.19	−12.79	1.28
			4500	133.19	−9.39	1.42
			5000	134.43	−8.55	1.5
			6000	154.59		2.58

Table 2.
Time optimization with variation of TR for SNR. T1/T2 608/134 (msec).

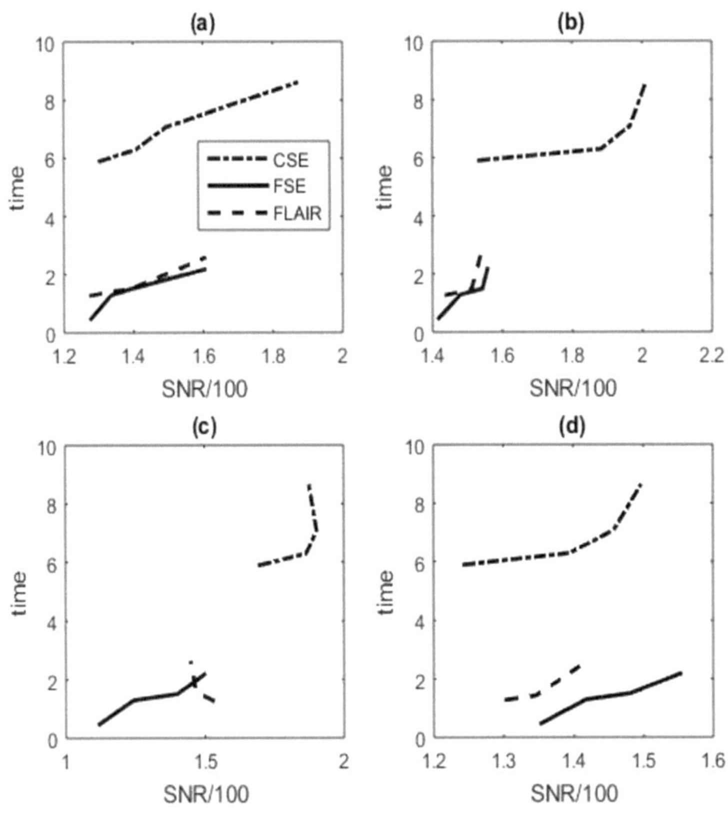

Figure 3.
Comparison between the pulse sequences for the appropriate SNR at short acquisition time (a) T1/T2 of the phantom is 608/134 msec. (b) T1/T2 of the phantom is 759/155 msec. (c) T1/T2 of the phantom is 917/135 msec. (d) T1/T2 of the phantom is 986/220 msec.

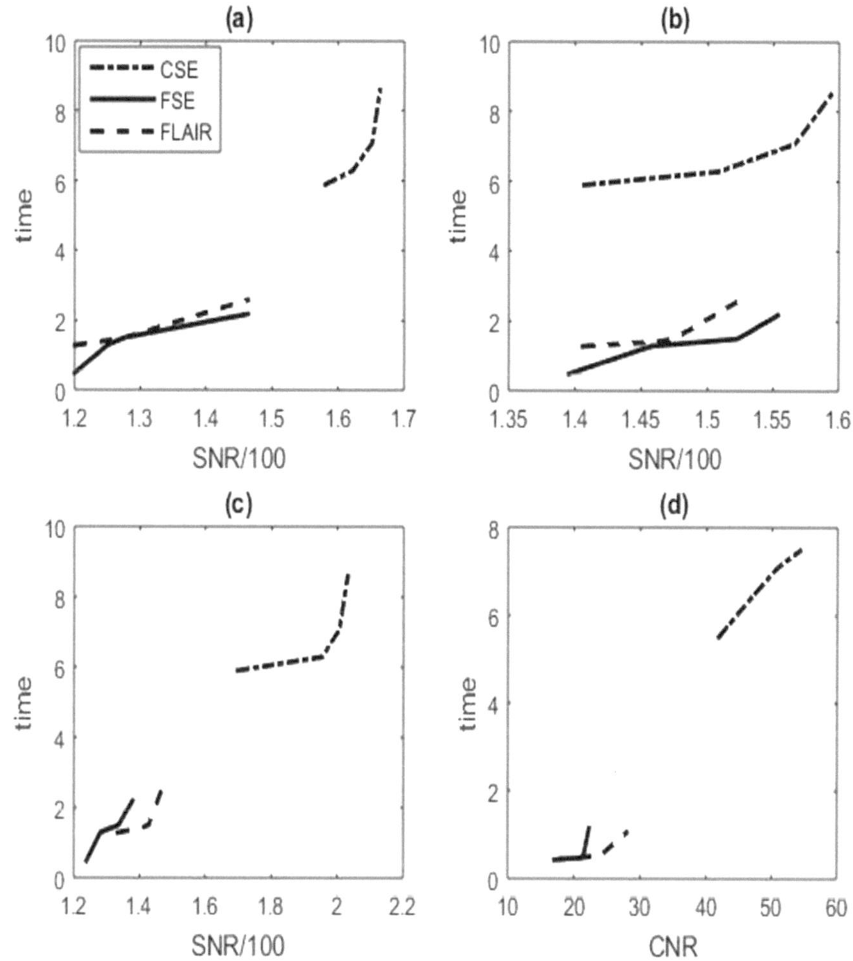

Figure 4.
Comparison between the pulse sequences for appropriate SNR at short acquisition time. (a) T1/T2 of the phantom is 1050/164 msec. (b) T1/T2 of the phantom is 1180/220 msec. (c) T1/T2 of the phantom is 1296/200 msec. (d) Comparison among pulse sequences for good CNR at short acquisition time,T1/T2 of the phantoms are 628/58 and 812/166 (msec).

T2-weighted images makes FSE more prevalent. For images with a good SNR, the FSE acquires data 79% quicker compared to the CSE (**Figure 3d**).

As shown in **Table 6**, the T/T2 time of this phantom is 1050/164 (msec), FSE and FLAIR created the image's SNR in the shortest possible period of time, FLAIR and CSE also provided a good image with the least amount of error for given values. FLAIR can be a good option for selecting various TR values because it has a quicker acquisition time than CSE. FSE and FLAIR have precise SNR of the image and acquisition times that are 63% and 56% faster than CSE, respectively (**Figure 4a**).

While FSE and FLAIR may be preferable in terms of the time of acquisition, as demonstrated in **Table 7**, the phantom's T1/T2 time is 1180/221 (msec); CSE, FSE, and FLAIR equally generate accurate SNR. To achieve an accurate signal-to-noise ratio (SNR) of the image, both the FSE and FLAIR pulse sequences require 76% and 77% less time, respectively, compared to the CSE sequence (**Figure 4b**).

Sr. no	Pulse sequences	T1/T2 of phantom (msec)	TR (msec)	SNR	Percentage error (%)	Acquisition time (min: sec)
1	CSE	759/155	1800	153.43		5.9
			2000	188.21	19.88	6.29
			2200	196.39	25.08	7.08
			2400	201.07	28.07	8.59
2	FSE	759/155	4000	141.78	−3.54	0.48
			4200	148.05		1.29
			4400	154.30		1.5
			4600	155.76		2.18
3	FLAIR	759/155	4000	143.99	−2.04	1.28
			4500	149.73		1.42
			5000	151.26		1.5
			6000	153.61		2.58

Table 3.
Time optimization with variation of TR for SNR. T1/T2 759/155 (msec).

Sr. No	Pulse sequences	T1/T2 of phantom (msec)	TR (msec)	SNR	Percentage error (%)	Acquisition time (min:sec)
1	CSE	917/135	1800	169.85	8.18	5.9
			2000	186.43	18.74	6.29
			2200	190.23	21.16	7.08
			2400	187.61	19.49	8.59
2	FSE	917/135	4000	89.48	−39.12	0.48
			4200	92.97	−36.75	1.29
			4400	96.79	−34.15	1.5
			4600	105.05	−28.53	2.18
3	FLAIR	917/135	4000	97.37	−33.76	1.28
			4500	102.25	−30.43	1.42
			5000	103.54	−29.55	1.5
			6000	115.05	−21.73	2.58

Table 4.
Time optimization with variation of TR for SNR. T1/T2 917/135 (msec).

Sr. No	Pulse sequences	T1/T2 of phantom (msec)	TR (msec)	SNR	Percentage error (%)	Acquisition time (msec)
1	CSE	986/220	1800	124.39	−15.64	5.9
			2000	139.46	−5.124	6.29
			2200	145.72		7.08
			2400	149.55		8.59
2	FSE	986/220	4000	135.31	−7.951	0.48
			4200	141.76	−3.561	1.29
			4400	148.07		1.5
			4600	155.30		2.18
3	FLAIR	986/220	4000	130.37	−11.311	1.28
			4500	134.51	−8.495	1.42
			5000	135.06	−8.115	1.5
			6000	141.75	−3.565	2.58

Table 5.
Time optimization with variation of TR for SNR. T1/T2 986/220 (msec).

Sr. no	Pulse sequences	T1/T2 of phantom (msec)	TR (msec)	SNR	Percentage error (%)	Acquisition time (msec)
1	CSE	1050/164	1800	158.06		5.9
			2000	162.18	3.30	6.29
			2200	165.16	5.19	7.08
			2400	166.33	5.94	8.59
2	FSE	1050/164	4000	120.02	−18.35	0.48
			4200	124.97	−14.98	1.29
			4400	127.54	−13.23	1.5
			4600	146.27		2.18
3	FLAIR	1050/164	4000	133.31	−9.31	1.28
			4500	139.82	−4.88	1.42
			5000	141.91	−3.45	1.5
			6000	159.56		2.58

Table 6.
Time optimization with variation of TR for SNR. T1/T2 1050/164 (msec).

Sr. no	Pulse sequences	T1/T2 of phantom (msec)	TR (msec)	SNR	Percentage error (%)	Acquisition time (msec)
1	CSE	1180/221	1800	140.68	−4.76	5.9
			2000	150.88		6.29
			2200	156.62		7.08
			2400	159.58	1.64	8.59
2	FSE	1180/221	4000	139.54	−5.06	0.48
			4200	145.79		1.29
			4400	152.29	−0.82	1.5
			4600	155.36		2.18
3	FLAIR	1180/221	4000	140.58	−4.36	1.28
			4500	146.24		1.42
			5000	147.43		1.5
			6000	152.34		2.58

Table 7.
Time optimization with variation of TR for SNR. T1/T2 1180/221(msec).

Sr. No	Pulse sequences	T1/T2 of phantom (msec)	TR (msec)	SNR	Percentage error (%)	Acquisition time (min: sec)
1	CSE	1296/200	1800	169.75	8.12	5.9
			2000	195.49	24.51	6.29
			2200	200.60	27.77	7.08
			2400	203.09	29.35	8.59
2	FSE	1296/200	4000	123.82	−15.76	0.48
			4200	128.08	−12.86	1.29
			4400	133.62	−9.09	1.5
			4600	137.85	−6.22	2.18
3	FLAIR	1296/200	4000	133.38	−9.26	1.28
			4500	140.73	−4.26	1.42
			5000	142.76	−2.87	1.5
			6000	147.13		2.58

Table 8.
Time optimization with variation of TR for SNR. T1/T2 1296/200 (msec).

Table 8 demonstrates that FLAIR is the only technique that can provide an image's SNR with the smallest errors and the shortest acquisition time (**Figure 4c**).

According to **Table 9**, T1/T2 628/58 (msec) & 812/166 (msec), the acquisition time of CSE in the T2-weighted study is longer than that of FSE and FLAIR. When compared to the FSE and FLAIR pulse sequences, the CSE sequence has a 144% and 94% superior contrast-to-noise ratio (CNR). CSE must be used for a long time in T2-weighted images to create a contrast between tissues (**Figure 4d**).

Sr. No	Pulse sequences	T1/T2 of phantom (msec)	TR (msec)	CNR	Percentage increase in CNR (%)	Acquisition time (min: sec)
1	CSE	628/58	1800	41.864	13%	5.51
		812/166	2000	47.292	7%	6.49
			2200	50.687	7%	7.07
			2400	54.267		7.48
2	FSE	628/58	3800	18.028	17%	0.45
		812/166	4000	21.147	2%	0.47
			4200	21.567	3%	0.59
			4400	22.283		1.14
3	FLAIR	628/58	3500	17.075	19%	0.43
		812/166	4000	20.331	19%	0.46
			4500	24.149	16%	0.54
			5000	28.002		1.05

Table 9.
Time optimization with variation of TR on CNR. Deliver dose 25 Grey & 0 Grey. T1/T2 628/58(msec) & 812/166 (msec).

4. Importance of acquisition time and comparison of pulse sequences

In clinical practice, the duration of acquisition is crucial in T2-weighted MRI imaging. The three most frequently used pulse sequences that are regularly employed at the clinical level for diagnostic purposes have been chosen. The idea of selecting the right sequence and optimising the experimental parameters to achieve image excellence at a quick acquisition time was shown by comparing these pulse sequences. Regarding FBX and polysaccharide gels, we assessed the CNR and SNR, respectively. We evaluated the performance of different pulse sequences by comparing SNR and CNR at the appropriate acquisition time.

Many options for TR in each pulse sequence were tested and researched in order to identify the pulse sequence with the most favourable combination for improved image quality with a respectably fast acquisition time. Each pulse sequence is usually exceptionally effective at selecting the right parameters.

SNR is a measurement of image quality. With an increase in TR, the image's SNR rises. The TR response is determined by the transverse time to the relaxation of a phantom object or biological cells [28] because T2 decay is caused by energy transfer between spins. To make T2 the dominant factor in the signal decay, a very long TR will be required. TR is a component that lengthens the process of acquiring the image. For the image's SNR and acquisition time to be maintained, an appropriate TR is essential. Image noise and contrast may become a limiting factor when TR is decreased to shorten the time required for image acquisition [29].

According to **Tables 2** and **6**, by considering the phantoms 608/134 (msec) and 1050/164 (msec), SNR of the pulse sequences CSE and FLAIR in the T2-weighted examinations are comparable. But CSE and FLAIR have quite different acquisition times. When compared to CSE, FLAIR's acquisition time is 63% and 56% faster. While other pulse sequences failed to sustain SNR at particular TR values, for the identical phantom, FLAIR covers a range of −33% to −21% while FSE has a percentage error between −39% and − 28%., **Table 4** shows that CSE is noticeably good for 917/155 (msec). For large T1/T2 weighting phantoms with an acquisition time of 1180/221 (msec), **Table 7** compares CSE to FLAIR and FSE, despite the fact that CSE has an acquisition time that is 372% and 398% as high as FLAIR and FSE, correspondingly.

In T2 weighted study as indicated in **Table 9**, the provided dosages are 25 grey and 0 grey, and T1/T2 values are 628/48 (msec) and 812/166 (msec) respectively, the signal intensity variation throughout the tissues is very significant. **Table 9** demonstrates the great disparity among tissues generated by the CSE at long TR. At the diagnostic stage, this pinnacle of quality in CNR is extremely appreciable and desired.

In MRI study, CSE's T2-weighted acquisition time is 556% and 612% longer than FSE, FLAIR, correspondingly; nevertheless, CSE's CNR is 144% and 94% better with TR selection. As a result, as illustrated in **Tables 2** and **9**, CSE must be utilised for an extended period of time to establish contrast among biological cells, in images that are T2-weighted.

As illustrated in **Tables 3** and **6**, FSE demonstrated very favourable outcomes for the phantoms of & 759/155 (msec), 1180/221 (msec). Similar to this, FSE for the phantom 608/134 (msec), 986/220 (msec), and 1296/220 (msec) in **Tables 2**, **5**, and **8** correspondingly show high SNR with low percentage error. As shown in **Table 6**, the FSE cannot be selected for the T1//T2 phantom of 917/135 (msec), the percentage inaccuracy is large, and consequently the SNR is very low for the phantom of 1050/164 (msec). The level of accuracy offered by CSE could never be matched by CNR in FSE. Because all the echoes were averaged into one k-space in the T2-weighted investigation, the adoption of a long turbo factor reduced the significance of FSE [30]. The MT (magnetization transfer), which reduces the contrast between normal and pathological tissues, also has an impact on FSE. However, by adjusting the echo factor, the contrast of the tissues can be adjusted [31–35]. In a T2-weighted investigation of FSE, optimal parameters are required to obtain improved CNR.

For a number of tissues, FLAIR and FSE are equivalent to one another in terms of SNR, and imagine acquisition time for tissues with T1/T2 time of 608/134 (msec) and 1296/200 (msec), respectively, as shown in **Tables 8** and **9**, FLAIR is an excellent substitute. The optimal TR selection improves CNR by 55% in FLAIR, which is often comparable to T2-weighted CSE. CNR for FLAIR has increased by 55%, however it is still 48% lower than CSE's. FLAIR has a strong tendency by employing TI (the time which relates to the null point of particular tissues), making an image contrast between tissues more visible by nullifying the signal for specific cells [36]. Images with poor inversion timing lack contrast between adjacent tissues. The inversion time and repetition time have a significant impact on the signal intensity differences of diseased tissues [13]. To get a strong contrast between tissues, the best inversion time is needed. These results underline the need for precision in determining the ideal imaging parameters at the diagnostic stage, in addition to the application of T2-weighted pulse sequences for certain tissue.

5. Conclusion of the comparison of different pulse sequences

In this study, we analysed factors within a pulse sequence optimally with the goal of obtaining image quality with a quick acquisition time. The correct TR value in each individual pulse sequence has a substantial impact on the precision of T2 measurement in MRI. It is clear from the results that CSE produced the highest SNR for a variety of tissues and produced a striking contrast in the images that are T2-weighted. Studies have demonstrated this, while the greater time required for acquisition seems less appealing, it does not reduce its utility in T2-weighted MRI studies. Despite the benefits of a quick collecting time and high image quality, FSE pulse sequence may be the best option once the obstacles connected with the complex interaction between imaging parameters and echo train length have been overcome. Regarding SNR, FLAIR is equivalent to FSE for a number of tissues. In a T2-weighted MRI scan, FLAIR images can also be advantageous pulse sequences with good SNR and quick acquisition times for different tissues. A pulse sequence with exceptional image quality in a quick period of acquisition was chosen as a result of comparing pulse sequences based on acquisition time. Indeed, a pulse sequence that offers excellent image quality and a fast acquisition period would be an ideal choice for clinical MRI. By combining high-quality images with efficient acquisition times, healthcare professionals can enhance patient care and improve workflow efficiency in a clinical setting.

Acknowledgements

We are thankful to the staff of the MRI department of Ninewells Hospital and Medical School, Dundee, UK for their support in collecting data and facilitating this research work.

Author details

Naima Amin[1]* and Muhammad Yousaf[2]

1 Department of Physics, COMSATS University Islamabad, Lahore, Pakistan

2 Mathematics Department, COMSATS University Islamabad, Lahore, Pakistan

*Address all correspondence to: naimaamin@cuilahore.edu.pk

References

[1] Lee HS, Lee YH, Jung I, Song OK, Kim S, Song HT, et al. Optimization of MRI protocol for the musculoskeletal system. Journal of the Korean Society of Radiology. 2020;**81**(1):21-40

[2] Hoinkiss DC, Huber J, Plump C, Lüth C, Drechsler R, Günther M, editors. AI-driven and automated MRI sequence optimization in scanner-independent MRI sequences formulated by a domain-specific language. Neuroimaging. 2023;**2**:1-20

[3] Esteban O et al. MRIQC: Advancing the automatic prediction of image quality in MRI from unseen sites. PLOS ONE. 2017;**12**(9):1-21

[4] Katarzyna K, Monika BF. Artifacts in magnetic resonance imaging. Polish Journal of Radiology. 2015;**80**:93-106

[5] Morelli JN. et al, An image-based approach to understanding the physics of MR artifacts. Radiographics. 2011;**31**(3):849-866

[6] Honda E, Sasaki T, Simms FC, Maruyama K. An optimized fast protocol for magnetic resonance imaging of the temporomandibular joint. Dentomaxillofacial. Radiology. 2001;**30**:126-130

[7] Tsao J. Ultrafast imaging: Principles, pitfalls, solutions, and applications. JMRI. 2010;**32**:252-266

[8] Morelli JN, Runge VM, Ai F, Attenberger U, Vu L, Schmeets SH, et al. An image-based approach to understanding the physics of MR artifacts. Radiographics. 2011;**31**(3):849-866

[9] Tsao J. Ultrafast imaging: Principles, pitfalls, solutions, and applications. Journal of Magnetic Resoning Imaging. 2010;**32**(2):252-266

[10] Tiago JG, Ricardo M. Advance in Ultravital Microcsopy: From Basic to Clinical Research. 1st ed. New York: Springer; 2014

[11] Mekle R, Laine AF, Wu EX. Combined MR data acquisition of multicontrast images using variable acquisition parameters and K-space data sharing. IEEE Transactions on Medical Imaging. 2003;**22**(7):806-823

[12] Augui J, Vignaux O, Argaud C, Coste J, Gouya H, Legmann P. Liver: T2-weighted MR imaging with breath-hold fast-recovery optimized fast spin-Echo compared with breath-hold half-Fourier and non–breath-hold respiratory-triggered fast spin-Echo pulse sequences. Radiology. 2002;**223**:853-859

[13] Naima A, Afzal M, Yousaf M, Muhammad AJ. Comparison amongst pulse sequences and imaging parameters for enhanced CNR in T1, T2-weighted study of MRI. The Journal of the Pakistan Medical Association. 2017;**67**:225-232

[14] Westbrook C, Kaut C, Talbot J. MRI in Practice. 3rd ed. Cambridge: Blackwell Science Ltd. University Press; 2006

[15] Ali CO, Ute L, Lena MO, Frank JR, Michael B. Comparison of ultrashort Echo time sequences for MRI of an ancient mummified human hand. Magnetic Resonance in Medicine. 2016;**75**:701-708

[16] Cheng L, Jeremy FM, Hamidreza SR, Hee KS, Felix WW. Comparison of optimized soft-tissue suppression schemes for ultra-short Echo time (UTE)

MRI. Magnetic Resonance in Medicine. 2012;**68**(3):680-689

[17] Michael PR, Kai TB, Hersh C, Jennifer F, Thomas M, Donal T, et al. Optimization of MRI turnaround times through the use of Dockable tables and innovative architectural design strategies. AJR. 2019;**212**:855-858

[18] Paul MW. A Test Material for Tissue Characterization in Nuclear Magnetic Resonance Imaging. London: Hammersmith Hospital; 1987. p. 213

[19] Medicine and Healthcare Products Regulatory Agency. MHRA 04133 Siemens MAGNETOM Avanto 1.5 T. January 2005

[20] Kelly RG, Jordan KJ, Battista JJ. Optical CT reconstruction of 3D dose distributions using the ferrous-benzoic-xylenol (FBX) gel dosimeter. Medical Physics. 1998;**25**(9):1741-1750

[21] Walker PM, Balmer C, Ablett S, Lerski RA. A test material and system alibration in MRE. Physics Medical Biology. 1989;**34**:5-22

[22] Afzal M, Lerski RA. Temperature dependence of spin-lattice relaxation times of ferrous sulfate gels. Applied Science. 2000;**19**:9-12

[23] Afzal M, Lerski RA. Time dependence of spin lattice relaxation time in Fricke gels. Applied Science. 2000;**19**:25-29

[24] Aalia N, Afzal M, Saeed AB. Effects of variation of MRI parameters on signal homogeneity: A qualitative analysis for ferrous benzoic xylenol orange gel. The Journal of the Pakistan Medical Association. 2010;**60**(6):470-473

[25] Afzal M, Lerski RA. Effect of concentration of ferrous ions on zero dose T1 value of dosimeter system. Applied Science. 2000;**19**:71-73

[26] Afzal M. Some Aspects of the Application of Fricke and Other Gels with NMR Detection to Image and Plot Radiation Beams for Tumor Therapy. UK: University of Dundee; 1998

[27] De Coene B, Hajnal JV, Gatehouse P, et al. MR of the brain using fluid-attenuated inversion recovery (FLAIR) pulse sequences. AJNR American Journal of Neuroradiology. 1999;**13**:1555-1564

[28] Carneiro AA, Vilela GR, de Araujo DB, Baffa O. MRI relaxometry: Methods and applications. Brazilian Journal of Physics. 2006;**36**:9-15

[29] Hashemi RH, Bradley WG, Lisanti CJ. MRI: The Basics. 3dr ed. Philadelphia, USA: Lippincott Williams & Wilkins; 2003

[30] Low RN, Francis IR, Sigeti JS, Foot KF. Abdominal MR imaging: Comparison of T2-weighted fast conventional spin–echo, and contrast-enhanced fast multiplanar spoiled gradient-recalled imaging. Radiology. 1993;**186**:803-811

[31] Siewert B, Muller MF, Foley M, Wielopolski PA, Finn JP. Fast MR imaging of the liver: Quantative comparison of techniques. Radiology. 1994;**193**:37-42

[32] Outwater HK, Mitchell DG, Vinitski S. Abdominal MR imaging: Evolution of a fast spin-echo sequence. Radiology. 1994;**190**:425-429

[33] Nghiem HV et al. The pelvis: T2-weighted fast spin-echo MR imaging. Radiology. 1992;**185**(1):213-217

[34] Catasca JV, Mirowitz SA. T2-weighted MR imaging of the abdomen. Fast spin-echo vs. conventional spin echo sequences. AJR. American Journal of Roentgenology. 1994;**162**:61-67

[35] Rydberg JN, Lomas DJ, Cookley KJ, Hough DM, Ehman RL, Riederer SJ. Comparison of breath-hold fast spin echo and conventional spin-echo pulse sequences for T2-weighted MR imaging of liver lesions. Radiology. 1995;**194**:413-417

[36] De Coene B et al. MR of the brain using fluid-attenuated inversion recovery (FLAIR) pulse sequences. AJNR. American Journal of Neuroradiology. 1992;**13**:1555-1564